The Chakra Experience

Your complete chakra workshop in a book

Patricia Mercier

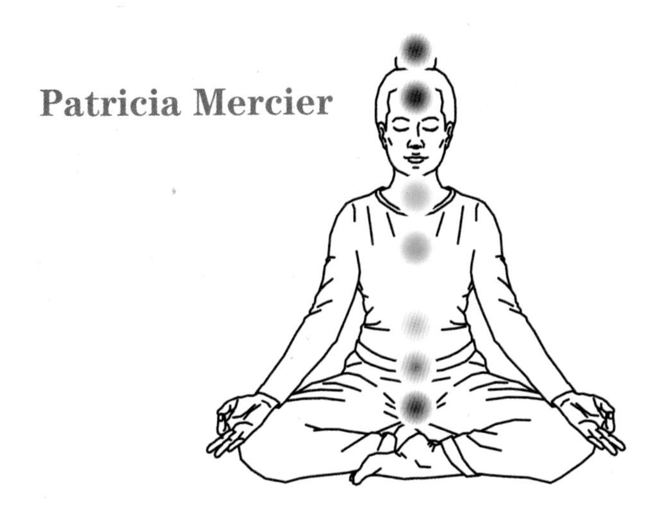

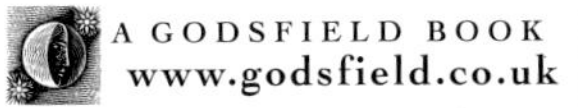
A GODSFIELD BOOK
www.godsfield.co.uk
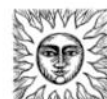

An Hachette UK Company
www.hachette.co.uk

First published in Great Britain in 2011 by
Godsfield, a division of Octopus Publishing Group Ltd
Endeavour House
189 Shaftesbury Avenue
London
WC2H 8JY
www.octopusbooks.co.uk

ISBN 978-1-84181-403-2

A CIP catalogue record for this book is available from the British Library

Printed and bound in China

1 3 5 7 9 10 8 6 4 2

Note

No medical claims are made for the information in this book and it is not intended to act as a substitute for medical treatment. In the context of this book, illness is thought of as a 'dis-ease' – the final manifestation of spiritual, environmental, psychological, karmic, emotional or mental imbalance or distress. Wellness and healing mean bringing mind, body and spirit back into balance and facilitating evolution for the soul; they do not imply a cure.

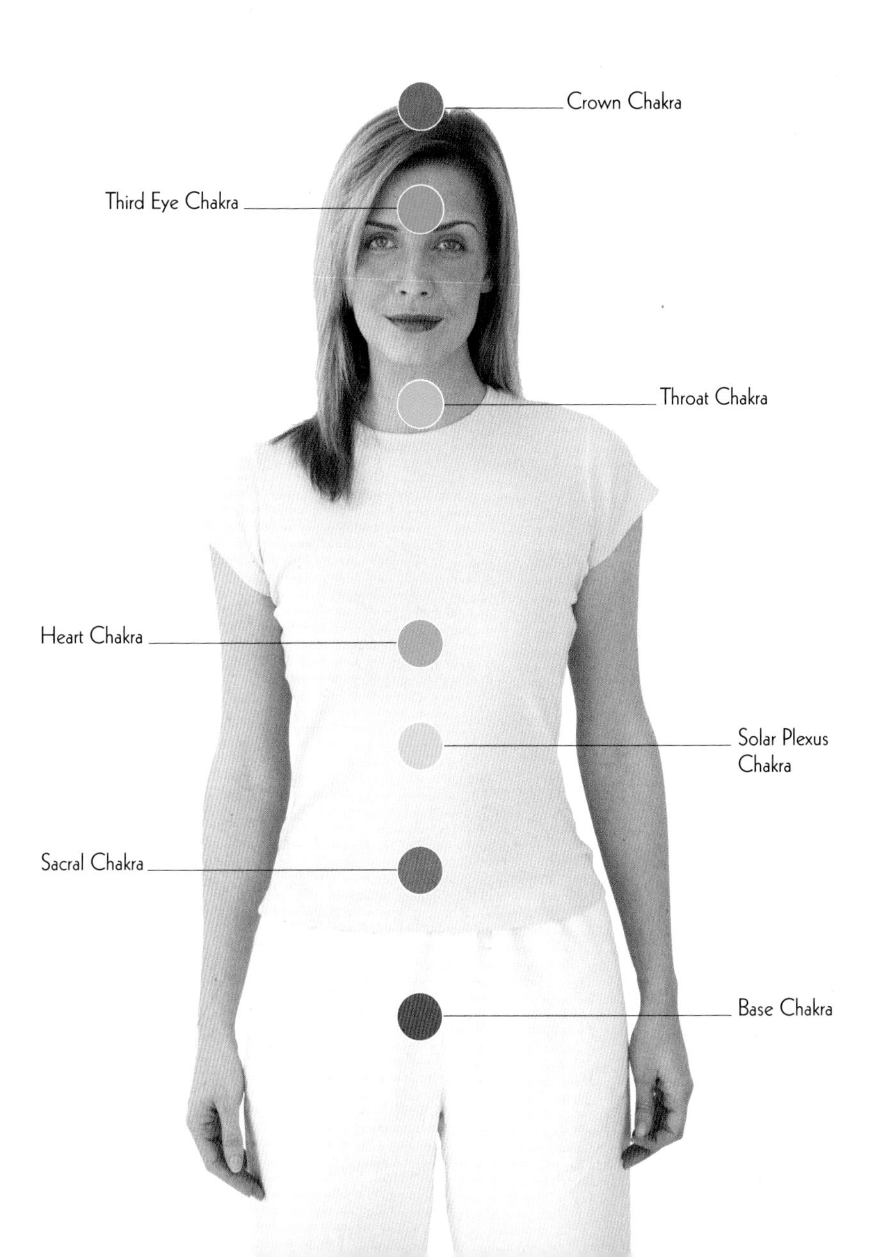
Crown Chakra
Third Eye Chakra
Throat Chakra
Heart Chakra
Solar Plexus Chakra
Sacral Chakra
Base Chakra

Becoming my own chakra healer

Using the knowledge in this book will help you take responsibility for yourself and understand what is right for you, by listening to the 'inner voice' that comes from your own 'truth'. It is important to be open-minded and to regard this as preventative 'medicine'. Dis-ease will always strike at the weakest part of your physical body. When you get in tune with your chakras, you may also activate spiritual development of a kind that does not normally conflict with religious thinking. The methods described in this book are core to holistic teachings and healing ways developed over the last 100 years, but draw upon ancient truths.

To experience your own chakras and become your own healer, you only need to develop intuition, heeding subtle messages from your body, mind and wider environment around you. There is nothing complicated to learn.

From my own training (first as a teacher of yoga, then as a holistic healer with colour, light, crystals, essential oils and Reiki), I have learned many practical ways to 'nourish' the chakras. You will discover them later in this book. *Give yourself quality time and space to follow them. Avoid being disturbed by people, telephones or excessive noise. Do not undertake the exercises if you are too tired.* If you approach this book in a calm manner, you will settle into a different way of looking at the world, giving yourself permission to relax and explore the mysteries of the chakras. Within these ancient teachings there is enough information for many lifetimes. Central to them is the knowledge gained over centuries through yoga and meditation, which open dimensions beyond your physical body. Understanding your chakra energies will give you command of your life and, most importantly, will bless you with time to be rather than *do*.

Work with your chakras now Turn to Exercise 1: Sensing and Drawing my Chakra Energies on page 34 and follow the instructions, before you read further.

Understanding the directional spin of chakras

People with auric vision usually describe chakras as having very soft and delicate swirling colours of light merging into one another, and sometimes spinning in a specific direction.

Everyone has a natural direction or spin to their chakra energies – either clockwise or anticlockwise. Whatever others may say, there is no right or wrong direction. This is a fluid situation and many factors can cause the natural spin to reverse temporarily. It may help healers/therapists to know that I use a pendulum to record the directional spin of incoming and outgoing chakra energies – and I do this both before and after a treatment. However, this is an advanced technique and does not feature in this book.

What I have discovered is that when the seven major chakras are harmoniously balanced, they alternate in their direction of spin from the Base Chakra upward. This is an ideal situation to work toward, using the balancing exercises in this book.

All chakras exert an attracting or repelling action, according to their direction. A clockwise chakra attracts an anticlockwise chakra, and vice versa. This is why we sometimes feel repelled by someone for no apparent reason – their subtle energies are just not in synchronization with ours. On the other hand, we are also drawn to some people as if they are an 'energy magnet'. This isn't surprising when we learn more about the chakras, for even our choice of sexual partner is affected by them.

We give off 'vibes' – energy messages – through our chakras to attract a partner. This occurs in both heterosexual and homosexual couples. During lovemaking a chakra ideally aligns with another of the opposite directional spin. So by balancing our chakras we are more likely to attract partners who are destined to enhance our auric energy field. In the future we will realize harmony in relationships and families is intrinsically linked to maintaining vibrant energy fields.

Are my chakras active or passive?

Some people describe chakras as 'open' or 'closed' – but if they were all closed, you would be dead! Better descriptions are 'active', 'underactive', 'passive/balanced' and 'overactive'.

Active means that your chakra is functioning well, maintaining a healthy input and output of the subtle energy known as '*prana*' (see the Glossary of Terms on page 251). When all chakras are active, your whole body and energy field will be vibrant.

Underactive means that your chakra needs help or stimulation – perhaps using the 'Energy Medicine' provided by the exercises in this book and on the CD.

Passive/balanced means that your chakra energies are resting or harmonious. This is the normal state to seek.

Overactive means that one or more of your chakras is functioning excessively to eliminate imbalances in your physical body, such as health issues. Sometimes overactivity aims to eliminate emotional imprints such as addiction, abuse or ancestral karma (see the Glossary).

There are two fundamental ways to influence your chakras and levels of pranic 'life-force', which in itself is usually a measure of well-being.

The first is by exposing your chakras to energy vibrations ('Energy Medicine') in resonance with the frequencies of a naturally balanced chakra. This can be achieved by means of practical exercises, using crystals, colour, light or sound, among other methods. Well-balanced *pranic* energy streaming into your body clears out the chakra like a breath of fresh air, and purification occurs. Sometimes this stimulates a 'healing crisis' (see the Glossary), but soon a deep sense of joy, serenity and clarity will enter.

The second way is to have the courage to just *be*. Take a decision and act upon

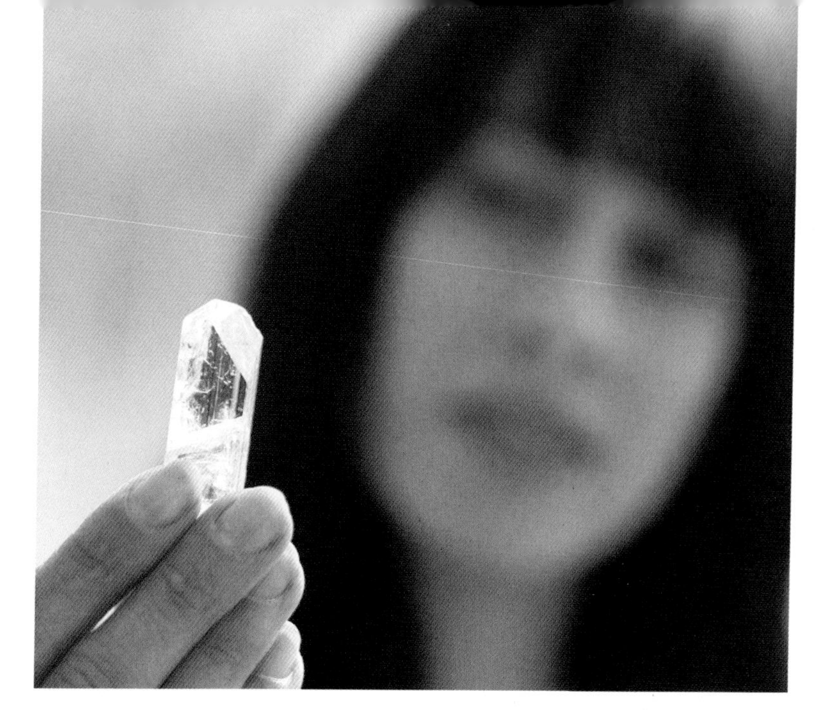

it. Key to this is relaxation, for unless you can relax, the auric mental and emotional bodies hold on to limiting ideas. Many people say they simply can't relax – even in their leisure time and on holiday, they never seem to stop their inner dialogue and never enter into an experience with their entire body/mind/spirit complex. If you recognize yourself in these descriptions, make an extra effort to undertake *all* the exercises more than once.

Work with your chakras now Turn to Exercise 15: Complete Relaxation on page 110, if you would like to learn a tried-and-tested relaxation technique now.

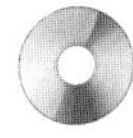

Work with the CD now Listen to CD reference Track 2, to hear the same relaxation technique being read out to you.

Using a pendulum

A pendulum is a very useful 'tool' for your work with chakras. Using a pendulum is not a party game – you need to take seriously the energies it shows you. Practise on your own until you develop empathy and get the hang of it. Pendulum 'dowsing', as it is called, gives access to all manner of information that the conscious mind would not have thought possible. The limitation is that you must formulate questions to which there is *only* a 'Yes' or 'No' answer. Please understand the need to disconnect completely from the outcome of the answer, since your mind or ego can influence the swing of the pendulum.

You may use a small jewellery pendant, a natural stone with a hole in it or even a heavy button as a pendulum, although you may prefer to choose a beautiful purpose-made crystal one. Ensure that your pendulum is well balanced and has a pointed tip. It is essential to feel comfortable with whatever you use, for it becomes an extension of your own subtle-energy field, detecting (among other things) slight variations in the surrounding areas that are normally not consciously picked up. If you have a crystal pendulum, wash it and dedicate it to the chakras, keeping it solely for your personal use.

How to hold the pendulum

Hold it between your thumb and first finger, from a chain or cord approximately 15–20 cm (6–8 in) in length. Tuck your elbow tightly into your body, and hold your arm and hand parallel to the floor. This keeps both hand and pendulum in the general area of the Solar Plexus Chakra and enhances the results.

'Yes' or 'No'?

To discover your reactions, relax, take a few calm breaths, then hold the pendulum a little above the palm of your other hand, and ask, 'Is my name...........?' (giving your own name). The pendulum should react immediately, swinging in a circle either clockwise or anticlockwise (occasionally it is a movement from side to side or front to back). This is your 'Yes' response. Run your hand down your pendulum to bring it back to a resting position.

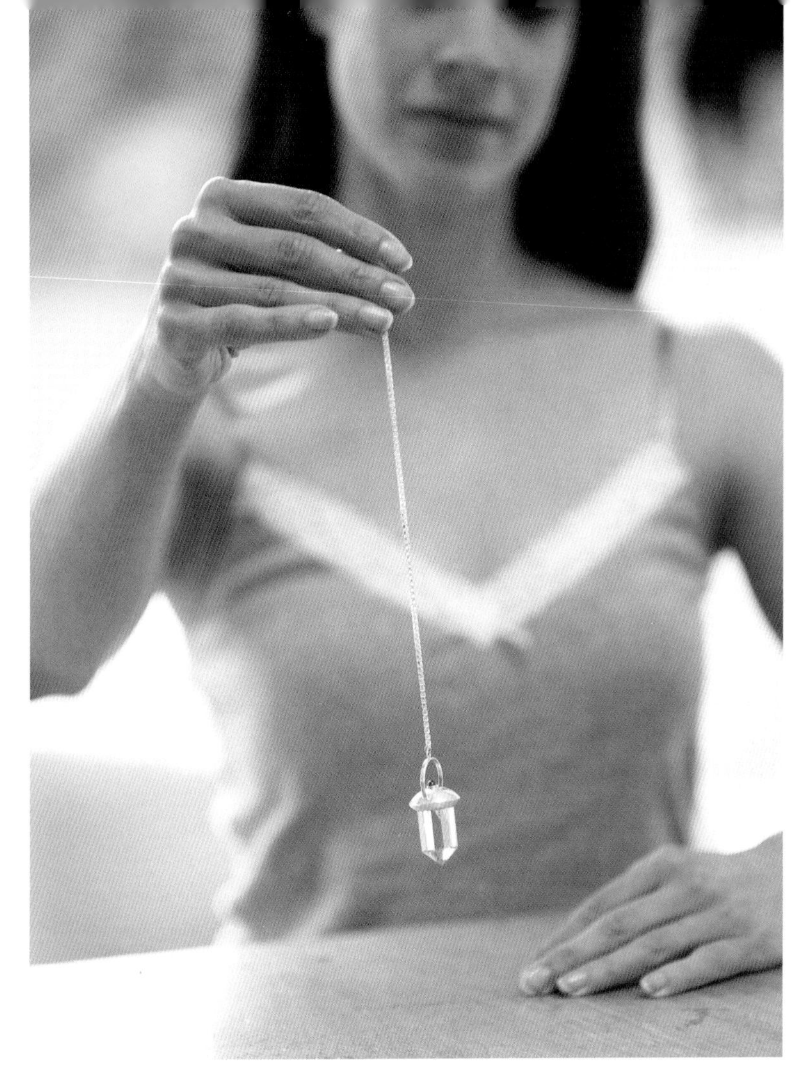

Now check your 'No' reaction. Ask, 'Is my name............?' (giving a false name). The pendulum should immediately swing in the opposite direction. Practise for a while, asking questions to which you know there is a 'Yes' or 'No' answer.

Setting up my sacred space

Your 'space' – the area your body/mind/spirit complex occupies – is already sacred. Problems with our energies arise when we forget this, and believe that we are separate from our environment or from our connection to the wider influences of the cosmic field of life and light.

To enhance your practice of the exercises in this book, it is helpful either to be in a harmonious natural setting or to create your own special place indoors. In both instances the sacredness within us – actually within our own 'innerscape' – and the 'outerscape' are one and the same, a reflection of each other.

Set aside a space inside where you will not be disturbed, in order to experience your chakras. Turn off the telephone, and every time you use the space, light a candle and some incense to remind you of the sacred Light. Play harmonious music or listen to CD reference Track 2. You may wish to make an altar as a point of focus, because it is a reflection of your connection to 'all that is'. You can create this using:

- Flowers, candles, an aromatherapy oil diffuser/vaporizer;
- Objects you have found in Nature;
- Photographs of your loved ones or the spiritual being/s who guide you;
- Offerings of bread, salt, food, water or other items that respect the traditions in which you were raised or that you embody today;
- Offerings representing the elemental forces of Earth, Water, Fire, Air and Spirit/Ether;
- Items or photographs representing positive aspects of your life;
- Prayers, poems or inspirational words to read out loud and focus upon.

Keep any crystals that you use for the chakra exercises upon your altar. Explain and share your altar with special friends and members of your family who are interested.

The elements

The elements of Earth, Water, Fire and Air resonate with the first four chakras. You can petition the elemental forces to help clear blockages caused by the stress of daily life – an indication of

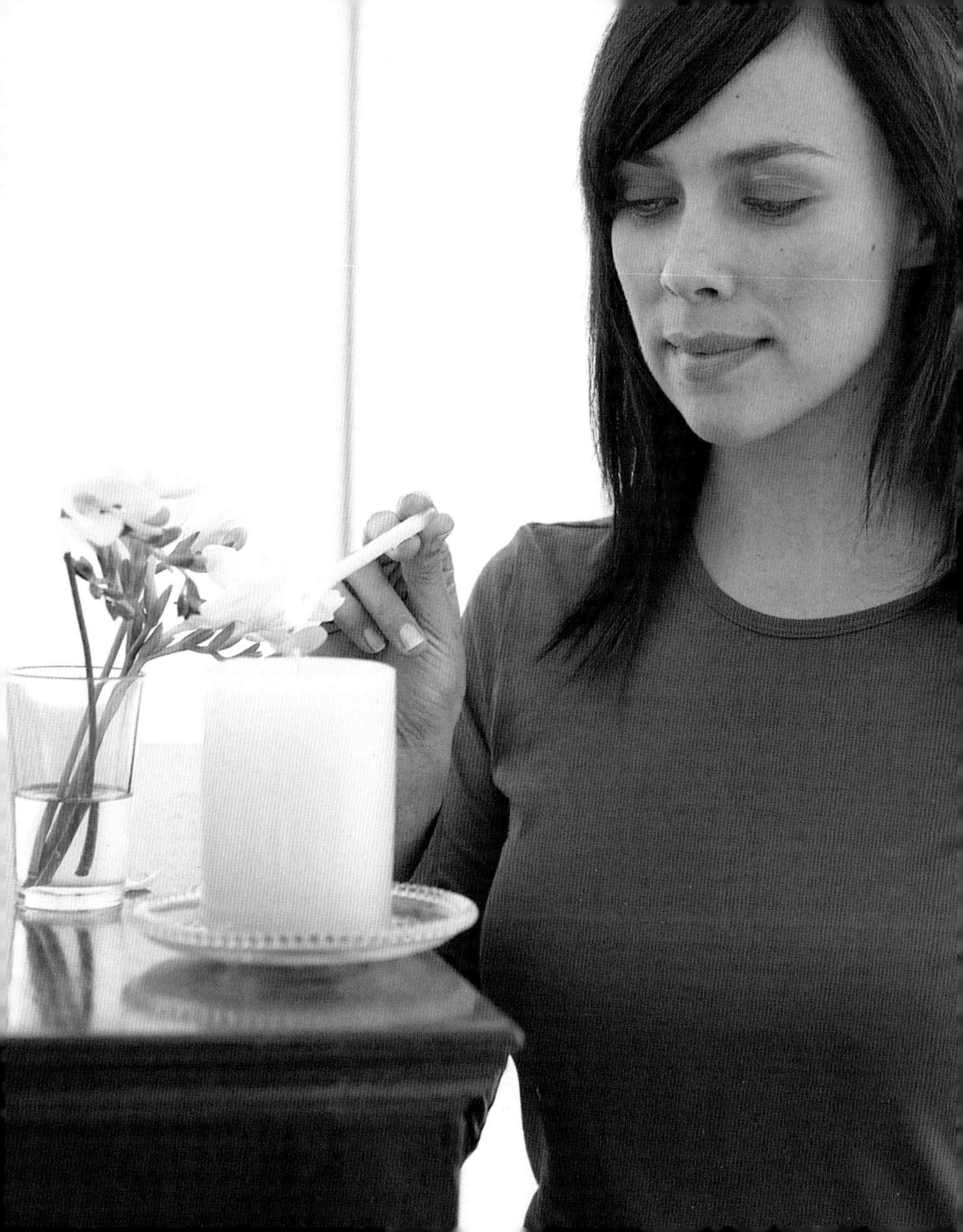

most people's alienation from Nature. Do not think of the elements as abstract ideas, for esoteric teachings have given them form as gods, goddesses or beings: devas/fairies, nymphs, salamanders and sylphs respectively. Above the Heart Chakra, the element of Ether is associated with the Throat Chakra, and Spirit with the Brow and Crown Chakras.

Work with your chakras now Once you have set up your sacred space, turn to Exercise 27: Candle Meditation on page 197, if you would like to learn a centring and visualization technique leading to meditation.

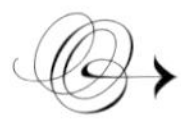

I'm not quite there yet Turn to Exercise 15: Complete Relaxation on page 110, if you haven't got time to set up your sacred space.

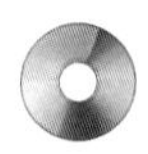

Work with the CD now Play CD reference Track 2, to learn how to relax completely.

THE BASE CHAKRA: MULADHARA

Work with your chakras now Before you read further, turn to Exercise 2: Sensing and Drawing my Base Chakra on page 38.

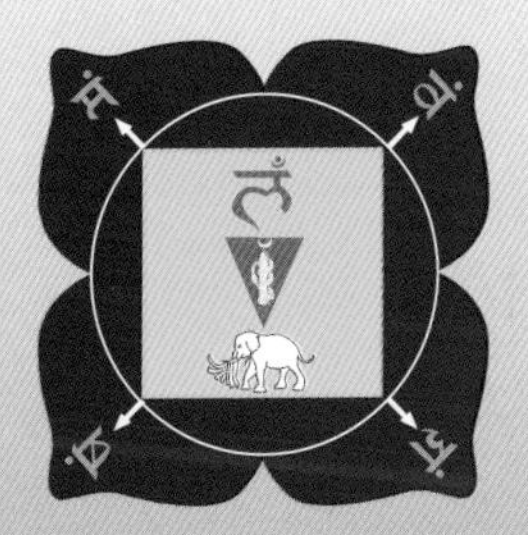

About my Base Chakra

Keypoints: Resonates with the Earth element and the colour red; concerned with sexuality, sensuality, survival and establishing a purpose in living.

The first chakra, the Base, is the source of life – it is from here that the physical body is established and grows. The Sanskrit name, *Muladhara*, means 'root or foundation'. This forms the vital foundation for all the other chakras, so you can understand why it is so important to balance the Base Chakra. This chakra initiates life through procreation and represents our will to live, maintaining existence on planet Earth. Red light, which is the lowest-frequency energy of visible light, stimulates this chakra. At the auric-field level the Base Chakra is linked to the secondary minor chakras in the feet, knees and gonads, and in addition energy flows to the physical body through the lower spinal area. Here are some ways to balance your Base Chakra:

- Relaxing and colour-breathing *red* light (stimulating) (see page 43);
- Relaxing and colour-breathing *pink* light (calming);
- Using crystals or aromatherapy;
- Enjoying healthy, uninhibited sex;
- Eating red-coloured food;
- Wearing red clothes;
- Learning yoga and mantras (see page 152);
- Exercising outside and appreciating Nature.

Work with your chakras now Turn to Exercise 4: Colour-Breathing Red on page 43.

Work with your chakras now Turn to pages 152–57 to learn about sound for the chakras.

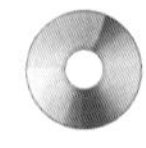

Work with the CD now Play CD reference Track 4 for a Sound Experience.

CHART OF THE BASE CHAKRA

Colour of influence	Red
Complementary light colour	Turquoise
Colour to calm	Pink
Physical location	Between anus and genitals, opening downward
Physiological system	Reproductive
Endocrine system	Gonads
Key issues	Sexuality, lust, obsession
Inner teaching	Establishing purpose on Earth
Energy action	Stabilization of Earth energy entering the body through feet and legs
Balancing crystals	Carnelian or 'grounding' stones under feet
Balancing aromatherapy oils	Patchouli, myrrh, cedarwood
Balancing herbal teas	Sage (in moderation), a detox tea containing ginseng or a mix of red clover, raspberry leaf, rosehips and damiana
Balancing yoga position (*asana*)	Virabhadrasana I (warrior), Trikonasana (triangle) and Garudasana (eagle)
Mantra/tone	LAM in the note of C (sounds like 'larm')
Helpful musical instruments/music	Organ, drums, double bass
Planet/astrological sign/natural House	Mars/Aries/first: life
Reiki hand position	Hands off the body over the genital area
Power animal (Native American tradition)	Snake/serpent

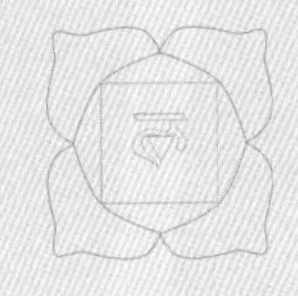

Body/Base Chakra connections

Each of the seven major chakras is associated with a point on the spine and with a ductless endocrine gland. For the Base Chakra these are the fourth sacral vertebra and the gonads (testes/ovaries) respectively. Disorders that affect the sacrum, the spine in general, excretion of body waste and the sexual organs are all connected to first-chakra imbalances.

Holistic health practice regards the person as a whole and looks for the underlying causes of disease, rather than the symptoms. It frequently makes a body/mind connection with the more subtle energies of the chakras. For example, chronic constipation could be referred to as a Base Chakra dysfunction caused by holding onto old, unnecessary thoughts and resentments, whereas repeating bouts of diarrhoea could again be a Base Chakra dysfunction, this time a reflection of rejecting ideas without assimilating them, due to deep fear.

Because the Earth element is assigned to this chakra, the best way to keep it in balance is to honour your connection to 'Mother Earth' and Nature. Try to take a walk outside every day and open yourself up to the beauty of your surroundings. Even if you are in a city, enjoy the sky, wind and sun. Seek out a park or some other haven of tranquillity where you might spot some of the creatures or birds that share the planet with us. Walk barefoot on the grass. Because the Base Chakra is your foundation, take a look around your home: is it attractive and safe to live in? Are there ways that you could improve its energy and ambience, for instance by treating yourself to a bunch of flowers or bringing the fragrance of natural aromatherapy oils into it?

'We tend the garden of Spirit whenever our chakras begin to open and as we strengthen our resolve to grow toward the Light. Like sunflowers that follow the course of the sun across the sky, we instinctively turn to light and move away from darkness.'

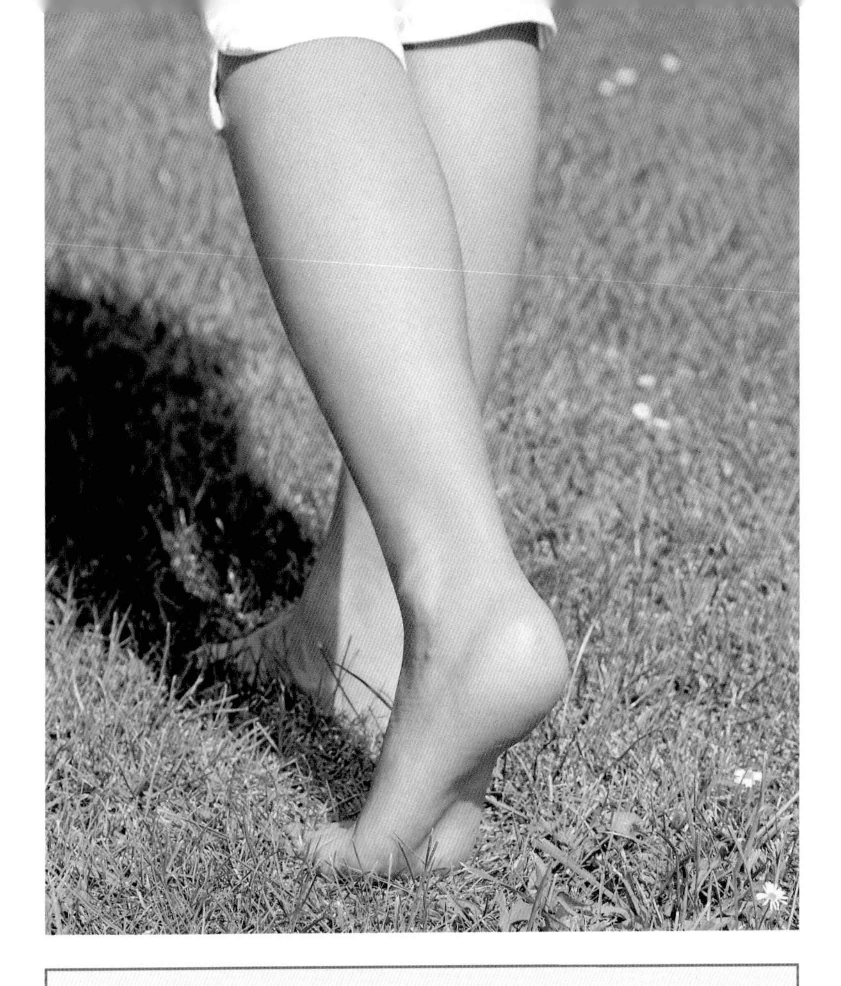

The benefits of grounding energies

When you are relaxing or meditating you might like to have a large stone under each foot, in order to ground what you are experiencing into the Earth Star Chakra beneath (an additional, newly awakened, transpersonal chakra, see page 220). Suitable stones are polished obsidian, iron pyrites or smooth pebbles from a river, garden or beach.

The energy of my Base Chakra

The Base Chakra, opening downward, draws Earth energy upward from the Earth Star Chakra (see page 220) to the feet and legs in order to process and stabilize it. This energy is channelled onward up the spine in a form that the body can handle, as signals that balance the release of endocrine hormones. Unfortunately, the first part of this process is often compromised and we fail to get the full flow of Earth energy. As modern humans, we have become out of touch with Nature by living in cities; by always walking on pavements in shoes and socks made from artificial materials; by buying de-natured food, instead of growing our own and having a relationship with the soil. The most likely and immediate health imbalance caused by alienation from our Earth Star and Base Chakras is persistent tiredness.

Have you noticed that, even in the most polluted, built-up cities, a few large trees manage to survive healthily? They have developed a strong root structure to feed them, which is as wide in its spread as the branches are above ground. Our 'roots', too, are energy connections that need to be strong and expansive.

Kundalini

Kundalini is primal life energy originating at the Base Chakra and normally dormant at the base of the spine. It is likened to a curled-up snake of sexual energy (or a strong *pranic*-type life-force in the Indian traditions). Kundalini is mentioned in the Tantric teachings of Vajrayana Buddhism. Intense sexual practices, such as Tantra, aim to move Kundalini up the spine by way of three major energy channels and the chakras. The central energy channel is called shushumna nadi, whilst the associated ida and pingala nadis intertwine all the way to the Third Eye Chakra. Tantric practitioners aspire to shift a burst of Kundalini energy upward, eventually to the Crown Chakra, where it unites with its opposite polarity, thus achieving enlightenment.

Maintaining the flow of Kundalini during lovemaking produces ecstatic

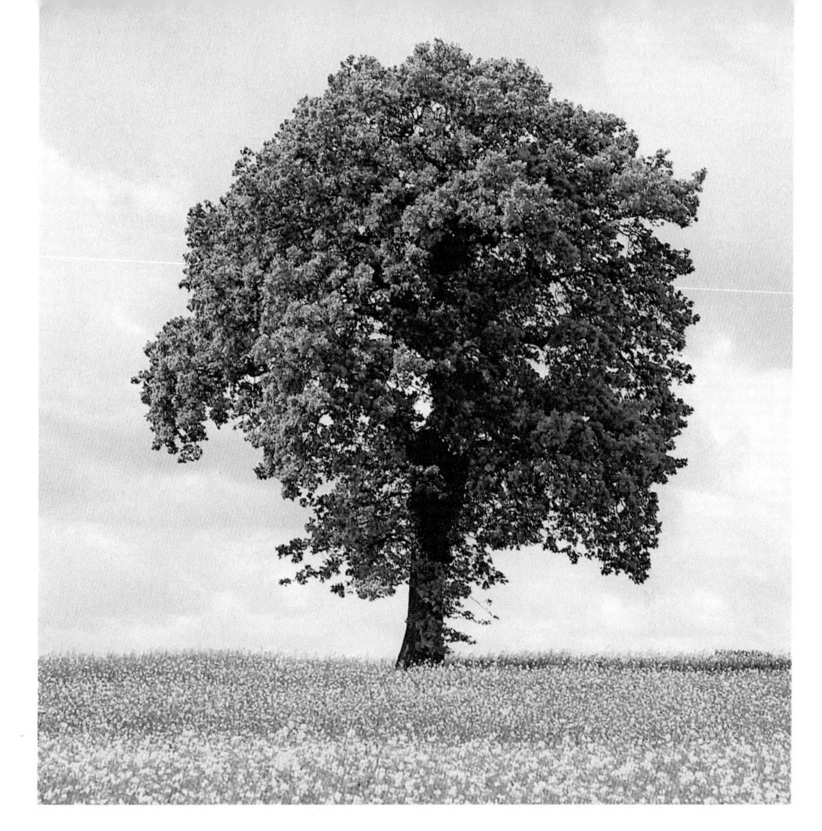

responses, which can be learned through ancient Taoist practices, including intense meditation (which is outside the scope of this book).

Imbalances

If you are unable to fully accept your own sexuality, Base Chakra flow becomes repressed and 'dis-ease' of the sexual organs may result. If you recognize that your fundamental lifestyle is imbalanced, your Base foundation will be imbalanced too. But take heart, for you can rebalance yourself in many different ways. The purpose of this book is to remind you that you can change – you can grow and flourish – simply by learning to be who you really are: ultimately realizing that you are a conscious soul having a physical experience and delighting in your body.

What influences my Base Chakra?

In our technological Western lifestyle, alienated from the world of Nature, we have largely relinquished responsibility for our bodies, in favour of medical intervention and artificial drugs. These are acceptable for supporting specific problems and life-or-death situations, and are administered with tremendous dedication and skill by doctors. But now we are waking up to empowerment through a preventative holistic approach to everyday healthcare. Chakras, body, mind, heart, soul and spirit are irrevocably interrelated. We can therefore choose to approach dis-ease in a different way, whereby a positive attitude of mind is vital. This is how.

Understanding the causes of dis-ease

First, consider what area of your body is affected. What is causing it not to function healthily, and what are the implications of the dis-ease? Explore the physical functions of the associated chakra areas: what is your body telling you?

Second, consider when the illness or dis-ease first manifested – what was happening at that time, and up to two years beforehand?

Third, ask: is this a recurring condition? Has a similar pattern, but a different dis-ease, occurred to me before, to family members or to close friends? Remember, too, that sometimes unwellness is just the process of letting go of old patterns.

Dis-ease may take a long period of time to penetrate the defences of your aura and chakras, before finally resting in your physical body. Natural holistic therapies also take time to clear dis-ease from your body, back out through the aura and chakras. Be prepared to work on yourself, especially on personal emotional issues, which may be the actual 'message'.

More than one chakra may be involved in imbalances in your body. To achieve results, always begin healing practices on the lowest chakra that is implicated.

What emotionally affects this chakra?

We will begin by looking at the message of dis-ease and at body/mind connections to chakras in general. 'Mind' is not just confined to brain functions, because there is an incredible connection between mind and body. With our body we express conscious thoughts and feelings through movement and action. So our body is the mirror of unconscious energies underlying everything we do. On the one hand, complex physical systems convey messages from mind to body; on the other, this is complemented by the intricacies of the chakras. Our bodies are a micro-universe interfacing with vast, converging possibilities. No wonder they sometimes baulk at the immensity of the task and we feel emotionally drained. Yet there is a need to personalize the question and ask: what is the message of this dis-ease in my body?

Every part of your body has a different message to give. You may say, 'I have to shoulder a lot of responsibility' or 'I am fed up to the back teeth'. Take a look at your 'body language' as you say these things. Are your shoulders hunched under too much responsibility, or is your jaw locked, with a habitual grinding of teeth to keep your despair within?

Here are some examples of Base Chakra imbalance:

- Leg tension and circulation problems suggest a holding-on, a lack of security and a disconnection with the Earth. Work on the Base Chakra and feet is needed.
- Imbalanced sexual attitudes may stem from abuse or fear. The key is learning to love ourselves as we are, and accepting that we can grow emotionally and spiritually, even from the direst circumstances.
- Lower-back, hip and pelvic pain all indicate closing down in these areas. We may require more honesty in our relationships, or need to understand that the universe will provide all that we require – but perhaps not all we want!

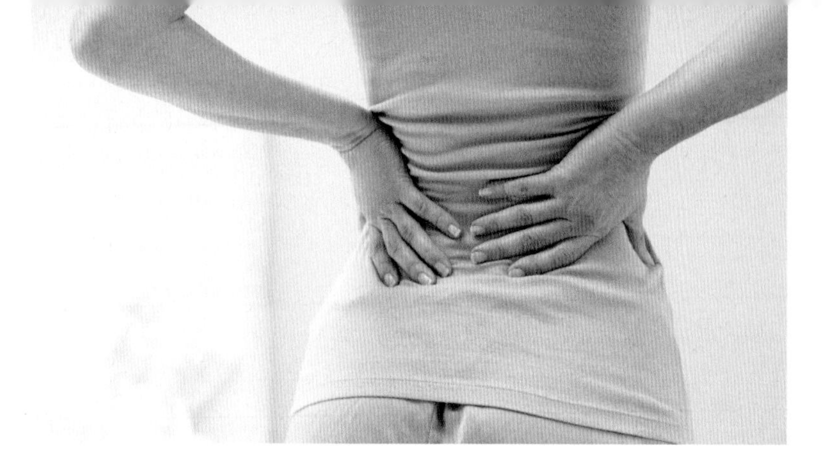

- Our joints are gathering points for energy and can easily block and stiffen – a reflection of our inner attitudes. Knee problems may arise from not accepting a given situation. They may lock with pain, but yoga and t'ai chi ch'uan movements will all work on releasing stubbornness or a fear of progress.
- Ankles and feet move us forward on our life journey. Dis-ease or stiffness in these areas represents conflict about going forward and accepting our direction. This is particularly true in issues to do with the home or with our developing spirituality.

Throughout this workshop-in-a-book you will find many ways to overcome limiting emotional states of mind. Have you ever been to a workshop that was really challenging – it will be the one you remember most, because no one promised you an easy ride? So remember that it is through life's challenges that we all grow. Many years ago my yoga teacher gave me a small piece of paper to study. On it was written: 'I am my own limitation. Without my own limitation I am.' Realizing 'all is perfection', gently accept or gracefully work upon limitations.

Work with your chakras now Turn to Exercise 3: Swallowing the Inner Smile on page 41.

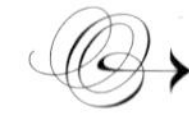

I'm not quite there yet Turn to Exercise 1: Sensing and Drawing my Chakra Energies on page 34. (There are additional body outlines at the end of the book.)

BASE CHAKRA EXERCISES

The following exercises develop the Base Chakra or Muladhara, which is the foundation of your being. Like the root system of a large tree, this chakra supports life, giving you your strength and drive. Because it resonates with the frequencies of red light you will learn how to 'colour-breathe' with the help of the CD, learn to smile inwardly, as well as learn to sense and draw the chakra energies.

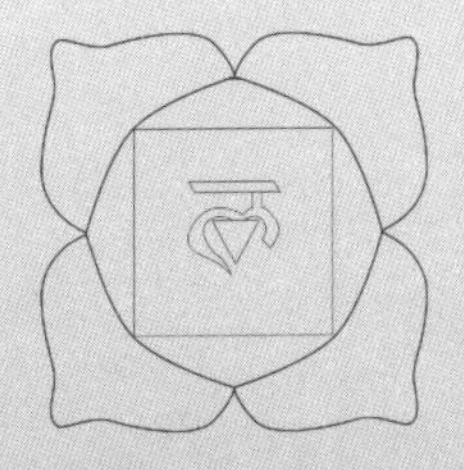

Developing intuition

Do this exercise before reading beyond this page. It will become a record of your subtle energy, to which you can refer back in order to chart your progress. This simple colouring-in of your body outline has been used successfully to train many holistic chakra therapists. It will enhance your intuitive powers.

Exercise 1 SENSING AND DRAWING MY CHAKRA ENERGIES

You will need: a set of coloured pencils or pens (all colours, including magenta, one of the high-frequency colours associated with chakras); keep the book open, ready to colour in the body outline opposite, which represents you (sign and date it before you begin).

- **To begin,** take five minutes sitting in a quiet place, breathing slowly, relaxing and closing your eyes. Now start to sense your body and your aura. Release any emotions that arise. Forget anything you have ever heard or read about chakras and auras. You are simply 'sensing' how your own unique energies are flowing at present. Check from your feet up to your head, to pick up any little clues that your body is giving you. Sense your auric energy field around you as well.
- **When you feel ready,** open your eyes and – immediately and without thinking – quickly colour in any parts of the body outline opposite as you wish. There is no right or wrong place to apply the colour: it is entirely up to you.
- **Once you have completed the exercise,** turn to pages 36–37 to assess your results.

My sensing and drawing my chakra energies experience

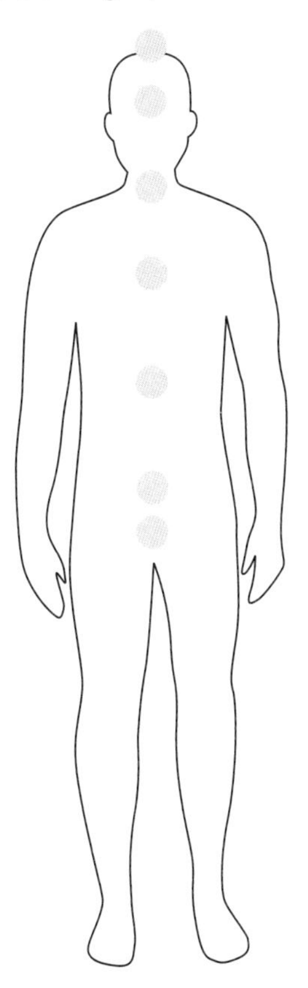

Date ______________________ Signature ______________________

Assessing my results for Exercise 1

Remember, there is no right or wrong way to have done this exercise, and there are no right or wrong colours to have used. To help you assess what you have drawn, here are some questions to consider:

- Have you placed colour on or near the chakras?
- Have you mainly used light or dark, heavy shades? What could that mean?
- If you have a pain or an issue with a particular part of your body, what have you drawn there? What colour have you used?
- Can you see areas where there is a concentration or a lack of colour? What could that indicate to you?
- Did you only colour within the body outline? Or did you use the whole page, thus showing your auric field as well?
- Look at your drawing carefully: are some parts of it strong and assertive, while other parts are weak? This is not a judgment, just a reflection.
- Look at the balance of your drawing from top to bottom. Is there more happening above or below your heart level? What could that indicate?
- Look at the balance of your drawing from side to side. Is your left side (feminine influences) or your right side (masculine influences) the strongest?
- Look at the feet – are they 'grounded', or is the body 'floating' and not connected to Earth?

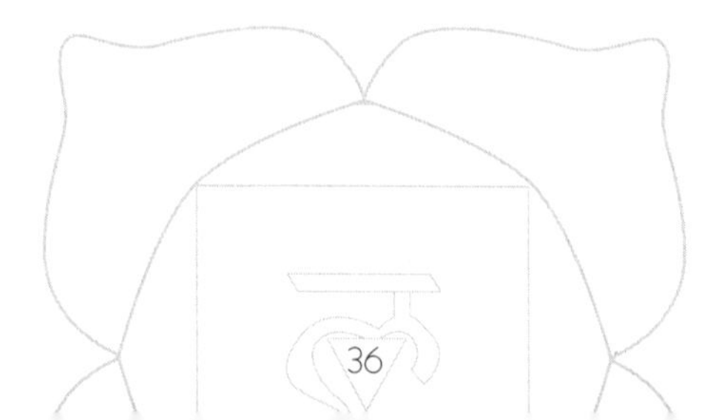

BASIC COLOUR INTERPRETATION OF BODY IMAGE AND THE SURROUNDING AURA

Is there a good balance of colour throughout? If not, ask why this is. Use the following guidelines to interpret your colouring:

Red Strength. Vitality. Or anger. Dull red in the aura = dis-ease or misplaced sexual energy.

Pink Unconditional Love. Excessive pink = ungrounded.

Orange Joyfulness. Balanced sexuality. Excessive orange = imbalance.

Gold/yellow Joy. Intellect. Mental processes. Excessive yellow = imbalance.

Lemon yellow Vitriolic personality/defensive attitudes. In the aura = change.

Leaf-green Balance. Dark green = moodiness, intransigence, unwellness.

Turquoise blue A very positive balanced colour.

Bright blue A very positive balanced colour.

Indigo blue Below heart level = heavy personality. Above heart level = dreamer/thinker/meditator. In the aura = sluggish energy.

Violet and purple Below heart level = ungrounded person. Above heart level or in the aura = spiritual development.

Magenta/ultraviolet A visionary spirit. But if in excess = need to 'ground' and work with the Earth.

Black Small areas of black in the aura or body = unwellness. At the feet = groundedness. Large areas of black = depression/repressed anger/addictions/dominance.

Grey Authority/control/repression. In the aura = unwellness.

Brown Similar to black.

Developing intuition further

Do this exercise before reading beyond this page. It is similar to Exercise 1, but will become a record of your Base Chakra – showing how grounded and realistic or how insecure you are – to which you can refer back in order to chart your progress.

Exercise 2 SENSING AND DRAWING MY BASE CHAKRA

You will need: a set of coloured pencils or pens (all colours, including magenta); keep the book open, ready to colour in the body outline opposite, which represents you (sign and date it before you begin).

- **To begin,** take five minutes sitting in a quiet place, breathing slowly, relaxing and closing your eyes. Now start to sense your body and your aura. Release any emotions that arise. Forget anything you have ever heard or read about chakras and auras. You are simply 'sensing' how your own unique energies are flowing at present. Check from your feet up to your head to pick up any little clues that your body is giving you. Sense your auric energy field around you as well. Now focus upon your Base Chakra area, from the pelvis downward. What is it 'telling' you? What can you sense? Does it feel free, flowing, harmonious? Or is an old pain or trauma held there? Does it feel 'grounded' – or have you shut off all feelings and thoughts of this chakra?
- **When you feel ready,** open your eyes and – immediately and without thinking – quickly colour in the Base Chakra area and any other parts of the body outline opposite as you wish. There is no right or wrong place to apply the colour: it is entirely up to you.
- **Read the interpretation** on page 40 after completing this exercise.

My sensing and drawing my base chakra experience

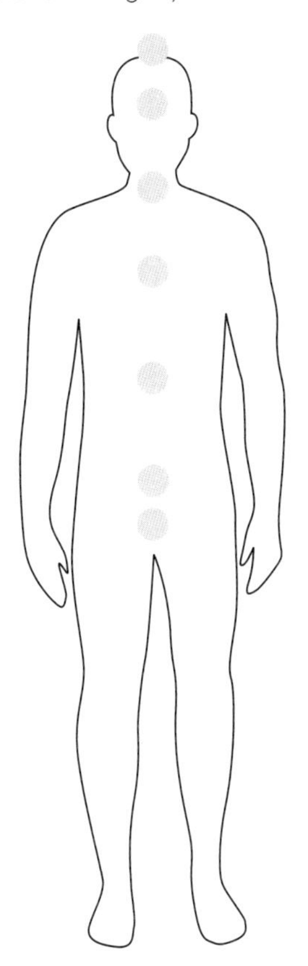

Date ______________________ Signature ______________________

Assessing my results for Exercise 2

A balanced Base Chakra will show strong and vibrant colours in the red/orange range. It will reflect trust in the natural flow of life, including your sexuality. It shows the basis of your health, vitality, flexibility, security and love for yourself and all beings. Balance here indicates being centred, grounded, realistic and able to take control of your life.

An unbalanced Base Chakra will show either very weak or very strong colours. These colours may be dark shades – black, brown or grey. It will reflect an attachment to material security, body-weight issues, pessimism and an inability to survive happily. Old childhood traumas are stored here, and weakness/excessive energy indicates low self-esteem, depression, repressed sexuality and fear.

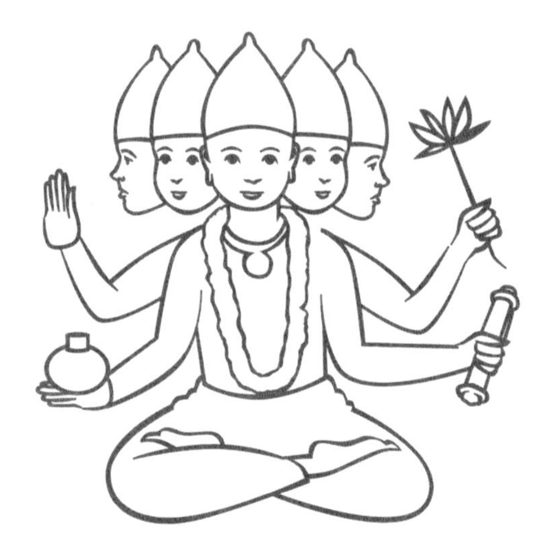

How to 'stress less'

The key to chakra balance is deep relaxation. Listen to CD Track 2 if you feel stressed or before undertaking other exercises. When any of the exercises in this book ask you to sit, use a hard chair with an upright back. Hold your spine straight, chin tucked in, shoulders back and feet firmly on the floor. Rest your hands on your lap, with the right palm on top, clasping the left palm. Breathe deeply through your nose with soft, long, smooth breaths right down to the base of the lungs – both in and out. This takes energy to your belly. Your tongue is a bridge for two channels of energy that flow through your chakras: hold it near the upper teeth over the palate. This prepares you for visualization or meditation.

Sitting as described above, you are now ready for the experience of swallowing your inner smile! This is an ancient Taoist practice and it will give you great inner strength and wellness.

Exercise 3 SWALLOWING THE INNER SMILE

- **The front line:** close your eyes. Allow an inner smile into your eyes, face, neck, heart and blood circulation, lungs, liver, kidneys, adrenal glands, pancreas and spleen.
- **The middle line:** feel saliva collecting in your mouth as your tongue continues to rest over the palate. Collect this saliva with your tongue, then swallow it down with a smile to your stomach, small intestine, large intestine and rectum.
- **The back line:** smile into your eyes, then down the inside of the vertebrae of your spine, from the top downward, one by one.
- **Open your eyes,** be gentle with yourself and with those you meet. Now record your experience in the space provided on page 42.

My swallowing the inner smile experience

Date ______________________ I saw ______________________

____

I felt ____

____

I learned ____

____

Date ______________________ I saw ______________________

____

I felt ____

____

I learned ____

____

Date ______________________ I saw ______________________

____

I felt ____

____

I learned ____

____

Tree visualization

This powerful colour-breathing exercise will connect you to your roots, which draw their sustenance from deep within the Earth, like the roots of a tree. You may record your colour-breathing red experience on the next page and/or make a drawing of your tree on a separate piece of paper.

Exercise 4 COLOUR-BREATHING RED

- **To begin,** sit in an upright chair or a cross-legged yoga posture. Ensure you are fully relaxed. Be in a place where you will not be disturbed for approximately half an hour – indoors is okay, but it would be even better to sit outside with your back against a large tree. Your spine must be as straight as possible and your chin pulled in, to straighten the back of your neck.
- **Close your eyes,** breathe slowly – visualizing your incoming breath as a vibrant red-coloured light – and deeply for a few minutes, focusing on the Base Chakra.
- **Be aware of the ground beneath you** (even if you are in a building) and start to visualize a strong root growing from the bottom of your spine and going into the Earth. Feel you are a seed that has the potential to grow into a huge tree.
- **See roots growing** from the soles of your feet, seeking out flows of water in the Earth. Be aware of tiny rootlets developing from your spinal root, anchoring you in the ground.
- **Now move to your trunk,** sensing that – like the main part of your body – it is a channel through which nourishment from the Earth can flow.

- **Check your body is finely balanced** on either side of your spine. Move on up into your branches. Imagine your neck and head, and perfectly balanced branches going out in the four directions: east, west, north and south.
- **Observe the shape of the leaves** on your tree; maybe there are flowers or fruit, or perhaps the branches are bare. Whatever you see, accept it.
- **Know that you have inner strength,** like a tree, that you can pull into yourself from the Earth. Thank the water and sun for nourishment, and the wind for its cleansing of dead leaves and wood in your branches. Know that you are connected to all other trees and life on this sacred Earth. Really, nothing is separate. All is One.
- **To finish,** start to breathe the red-coloured light more deeply. Reach down to your feet and rub them, then your legs. Finally stand up and stretch 'as tall as a tree'.
- **Now consider** the questions on page 45.

My colour-breathing red experience

Date ______________________ Signature ______________________

Circle the relevant answers below:

How well did I relax? Well / With difficulty / I couldn't relax at all

Did the colour-breathing help me focus on my Base Chakra? Yes / No / A bit, but then I lost the focus / Don't know

Did you see a tree? Yes / No

What kind of tree was it? ______________________

Was it strong / tall / large / small/weak?

Did it have a large trunk / a flexible trunk / a thin trunk?

Did it have leaves? Yes / No

Did it have buds or flowers? Yes / No

Describe them ______________________

____

Did it have seeds? Yes / No

How did this exercise affect me? ______________________

____

What have I learned from this experience? ______________________

____

Does my Base Chakra feel more balanced? Yes / No / A bit / Don't know

Pendulum dowsing

This exercise in pendulum dowsing builds up empathy and confidence with your pendulum, so that you can use it reliably to determine degrees of activity in your chakras. Avoid holding the pendulum over a chakra, particularly if it is a crystal pendulum; instead, point a finger of the other hand toward and near the chakra – this ensures that the pendulum does not falsify the reading.

Exercise 5 DOWSING MY CHAKRAS

You will need: a pendulum, and a pen to record your results.

- **To begin,** remain focused and silent for a moment. Then work systematically through each chakra, beginning with the Base Chakra and asking: 'Does this .... Chakra require balancing?' It is also relevant to ask: 'Is this .... Chakra overactive?' or 'Is this .... Chakra underactive?'
- **Record your pendulum results** on page 48 (date and sign your record), so that you can begin to see repeating (or varying) patterns of chakra activity. You may dowse just the Base Chakra, or you have space there to record the condition of all your chakras, if you wish. You can also compare the effects that various methods described in this book have upon your chakras, by dowsing before and after any balancing.
- **As an optional method of dowsing,** use a blank 'body outline' as given at the end of this book (see pages 238–49). Sign it (this is your 'witness' or energy imprint). With the understanding that this body outline represents you, rest your index finger on each chakra in turn. Hold the pendulum in the other hand, well away from your physical body. Ask the questions given above. Record your results on the following page, remembering to put the date on it.

- **Don't be concerned** if you can't immediately get reliable results. For some people, dowsing can take a long time to learn – particularly if the mind gets in the way! Continue practising another day, when your energy will be different, and eventually you will succeed. Helpful hint: don't look at the pendulum as you dowse.

Later, when you feel ready to do so, you may also work on the Base Chakra with any of the other balancing methods mentioned on other pages of this book. Consult the chart on page 25 to ascertain which aromatherapy oil to use, which yoga postures, colour breathing, and so on.

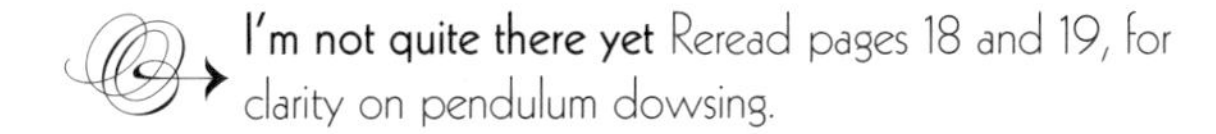

I'm not quite there yet Reread pages 18 and 19, for clarity on pendulum dowsing.

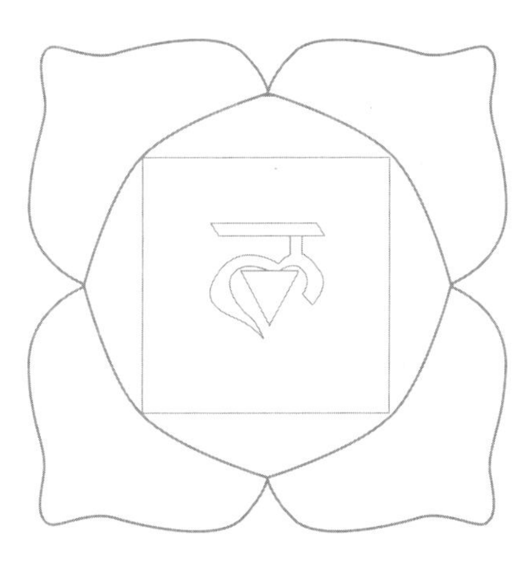

My dowsing my chakras experience

Date ______________________ Signature ______________________

- Does this ____________ Chakra require balancing? Yes / No
- Is balance required on a physical level? Yes / No
- Is balance required on a mental/emotional level? Yes / No
- Is balance required on an energy level in my auric field? Yes / No
- Is this ____________ Chakra overactive? Yes / No
- Is colour-breathing required? Yes / No
- Is crystal balancing required? Yes / No
- Is a change in my lifestyle required? Yes / No
- Is this ____________ Chakra underactive? Yes / No
- Is colour-breathing required? Yes / No
- Is crystal balancing required?
- Is a change in my lifestyle required? Yes / No
- Ask any other questions that you wish to pose.

Circle the relevant states below:

Base Chakra	Balanced	Underactive	Overactive
Sacral Chakra	Balanced	Underactive	Overactive
Solar Plexus Chakra	Balanced	Underactive	Overactive
Heart Chakra	Balanced	Underactive	Overactive
Throat Chakra	Balanced	Underactive	Overactive
Third Eye Chakra	Balanced	Underactive	Overactive
Crown Chakra	Balanced	Underactive	Overactive

THE SACRAL CHAKRA: SVADISTHANA

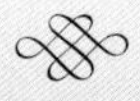

Work with your chakras now Before you read further, turn to Exercise 6: Sensing and Drawing my Sacral Chakra on page 66.

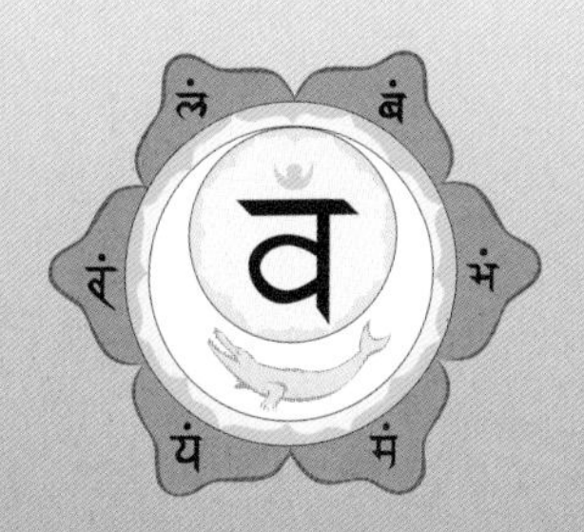

About my Sacral Chakra

Keypoints: Resonates with the Water element and the colour orange; concerned with sexuality, sensuality, emotions, karma and relationships.

The second chakra, the Sacral, is your vitality centre – flexibility here lets you feel content in your own body. The Sanskrit name, *Svadisthana*, means 'one's own abode'.

This chakra comes into play during puberty. It is responsive to the cycles of the moon and balances women's 'moon times'. A harmonious Sacral Chakra moves energy up from the Base Chakra to create sensual sensitivity and joy. It gives us fluidity in our actions, the ability to let go and express ourselves through dance, music and other creative arts.

However, if it is unbalanced, we may deprive ourselves of joy or spontaneity. It's not so much our feelings that will ebb and flow with this chakra, but our response to them. Unpleasant feelings aren't bad – they just need to be worked through and, if severe, may need professional assistance. Our vitality centre is watery by nature and is subject to mood swings, yet it is only by embracing our darker, more difficult side that we grow. And if we do not grow through adversity, then our inner child (see Glossary of Terms, page 251) becomes stuck at second-chakra level and we are unable to move energy up to other levels.

So allow time for recreation, non-competitive sport/exercise, play and laughter. Enjoy playing make-believe with children – they are great teachers because many of them remember who they really are at soul level.

In humanity's present collective incarnation, karma is an outdated attachment to time, causing compliance with archaic control mechanisms that rob us of our true inheritance as beings of Light having a physical experience – not only in this life, but in future lives too.

Orange light stimulates this chakra. At the auric-field level the Sacral Chakra is linked to secondary minor chakras in the groin and behind the knee, which are close to waste-removing lymph nodes. It is also linked to two minor spleen chakras.

CHART OF THE SACRAL CHAKRA

Colour of influence	Orange
Complementary light colour	Blue
Colour to calm	Blue
Physical location	Upper part of sacrum, below navel
Physiological system	Genitourinary
Endocrine system	Adrenals
Key issues	Relationships, emotions, addictions
Inner teaching	Seeking meaningful relationships with all life forms
Energy action	Transmutes sexual energy
Balancing crystals	Moonstone/aquamarine
Balancing aromatherapy oils	Sandalwood/jasmine/rose/ylang-ylang
Balancing herbal teas	Mix of spearmint, chamomile, liquorice, cleavers, corn silk and horsetail
Balancing yoga position (*asana*)	Parivrtta trikonasana (twisting triangle), Utthita parsvakonasana (extended lateral), Natarajasana (pose of Shiva)
Mantra/tone	VAM in note of D (sounds like 'varm')
Helpful musical instruments/music	Viola, lute, chords played on a guitar
Planet/astrological sign/natural House	Mercury and Venus/Gemini and Taurus/third: Education and second: Possessions
Reiki hand position	Two palms over the belly, then lift the hands off and place two palms below the navel
Power animal (Native American tradition)	Dolphins

Body/Sacral Chakra connections

The Sacral Chakra, also called the Navel Centre, is associated with the first lumbar vertebra and with the ductless adrenal endocrine glands above each kidney. Disorders that affect the bladder, kidneys, intestinal complaints and circulatory problems as well as the reproductive organs are all connected to Second Chakra imbalances.

The Sacral Chakra is concerned with assimilation, both in the sense of digestion of food and ideas, which bring about a natural sense of joy. When unrepressed, this produces a strong creative urge. This chakra is where sexuality is transmuted into the creative arts through self-expression.

Holistic health practice makes a body/mind connection with the more subtle energies of the Sacral Chakra. For example, because the adrenals release adrenaline at critical and stressful moments, the 'flight or fight' response is activated: we cannot decide whether to get up and run, or stand our ground and fight, so issues of self-survival are key. Closely linked to this area is the spleen, which supports (among other things) the production of immune cells in the blood. It is known that negative emotions impinge upon our body functions and the spleen is no exception, because anger particularly affects it.

Male and female concerns

Sexual dysfunction, such as sterility, may be concerned with hidden fears about having children, responsibility, financial worries or past traumas from our own childhood. Prostate problems in men are related to the sense of sexual power and performance. So, like women approaching middle age or the 'golden years', men too would be advised to move energy upward creatively through the higher chakras in order to relax in the fullness of older life.

Gynaecological or breast problems may be closely linked to feelings that a mother has when her children leave home. Her life had centred on the family,

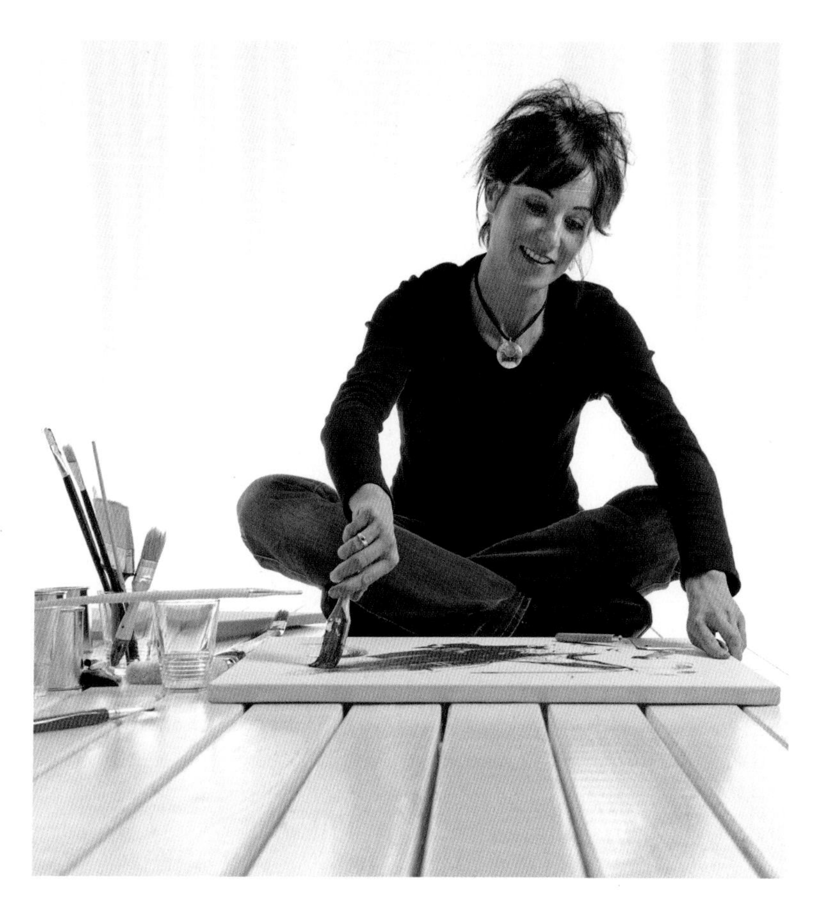

but then alternative interests are needed, which move the emphasis of her energies up from the Sacral and Heart Chakras onto other levels of understanding and into a time of personal spiritual growth.

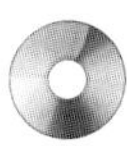

Work with the CD now Listen to CD reference Track 2 to help you relax, if you are feeling stressed.

The energy of my Sacral Chakra

The energy of the Sacral Chakra is softer and more 'feminine' than the strongly 'masculine' drive of the Base Chakra. It is the source of vitality for our etheric/auric body and the fountain of our passion for all of life – not just sexuality. It is the centre that leads us on to achieve marvellous things, triumphing over adversity and feeling happy and content in the process.

If your Sacral Chakra energy is imbalanced, you may ignore your feelings, disconnect from your sensuality and simply be too engrossed in your mind, living an ascetic life. Ask yourself the following questions:

- Do I celebrate my life and my accomplishments?
- Do I look after my body?
- Do I eat healthily and get enough sleep?
- Do I express my feelings?
- Do I take the time to look nice?
- Do I smile often?
- Do I sing or dance?
- Do I give and receive gracefully?
- Do I have a fulfilling sex life?
- Do I channel my life-force into creative pursuits?
- Do I regularly give myself a 'day out of time' just to relax?
- Do I exercise enough?

If you answered 'No' to one or two of these questions, then your vitality is weakened. If you answered 'No' to five or more of these questions, then your vitality is imbalanced. And if you answered 'No' to seven or more of these questions, your imbalance needs to be corrected: turn to page 41 immediately and do Exercise 3: Swallowing the Inner Smile.

Later on undertake more than once the exercises that you find particularly helpful in this book, until you feel you are achieving your full potential as a vibrant radiant being.

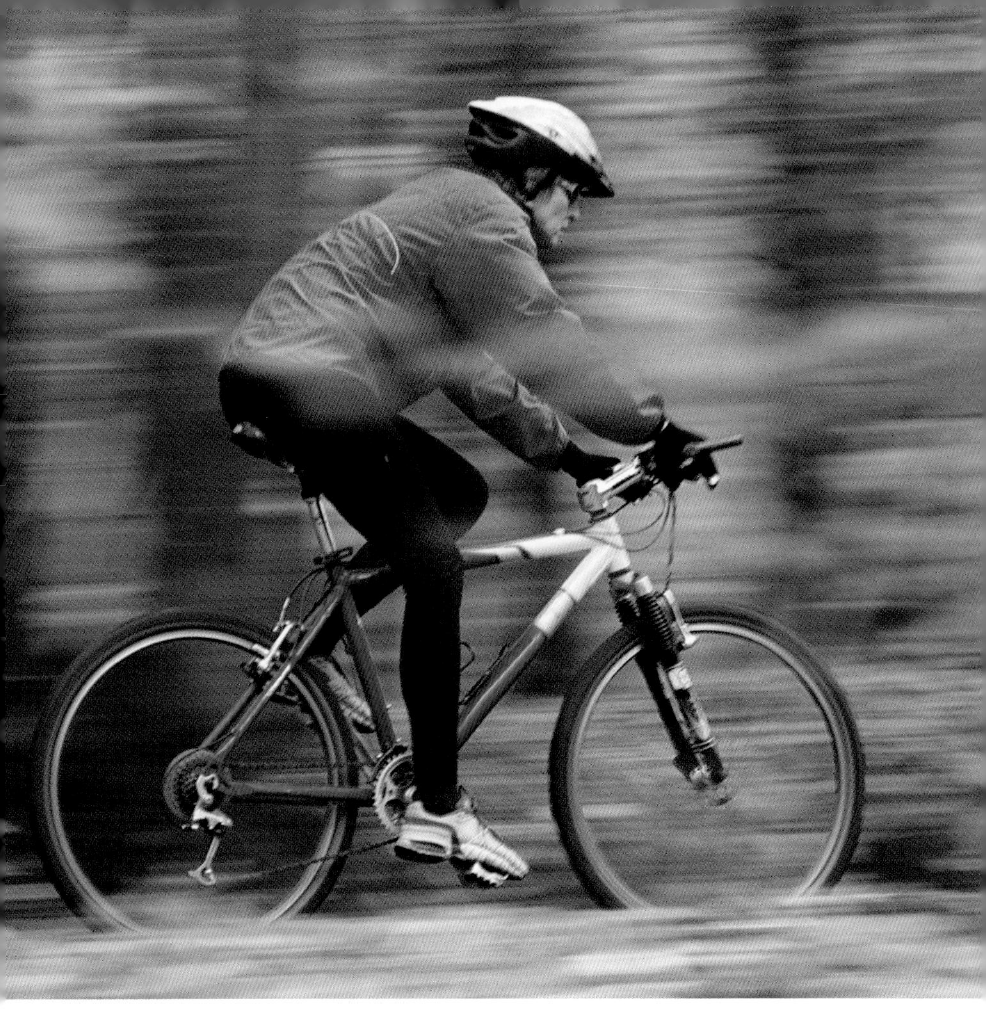

Work with your chakras now Turn to Exercise 8: Dowsing my Sacral Chakra on page 73, to check that your Sacral Chakra is balanced.

Work with your chakras now Turn to Exercise 9: Using Crystals on page 75, to balance your Sacral Chakra.

What influences my Sacral Chakra?

The element of Water is associated with the genitourinary system and influences the Sacral Chakra. Our sense of taste is linked to this chakra. It is well known that the moon controls the flow of all liquids on the Earth, and in us! The water we take into our bodies is beneficially encoded with an imprint of cosmic forces transduced through the moon. Even our hormones respond to the flow of tides, the phases of the moon and psychic changes that occur as waves of life experience.

Watery remedies

Because the Water element is assigned to Svadisthana, balance it by enjoying your connection to 'Mother Earth', the moon and Nature. Try to swim often. Drink sufficient pure water; increase your intake of salad foods and orange-coloured fruits and vegetables, because their water and mineral content cleanses the body. Create your own spa by giving yourself a few hours of luxury. Start with a mud or seaweed face-pack, then take a long, hot soak in a bath with mineral salts (or sea salt if you cannot get genuine mineral salts). Finish with a cool shower and pamper yourself with your favourite body lotion.

If this chakra is underactive there will be an urge to overindulge in food or sex as compensation, causing obesity, food intolerances, chronic skin conditions or possibly even impotence, sexual cravings and disease. Overactivity will lead to confused sexuality, unless it is balanced by the influence of the Heart Chakra. These effects are the physical body making its demands known. *Listen to your body;* take notice of any early symptoms it communicates to you. Even talk back to your body, telling it what you are doing to help yourself. Have a conversation with each of your chakras in turn, asking them what they need – unless you ask, you will never know!

Work with your chakras now Turn to Exercise 10: Colour-Breathing a Rainbow on page 77, to begin to balance all your chakras.

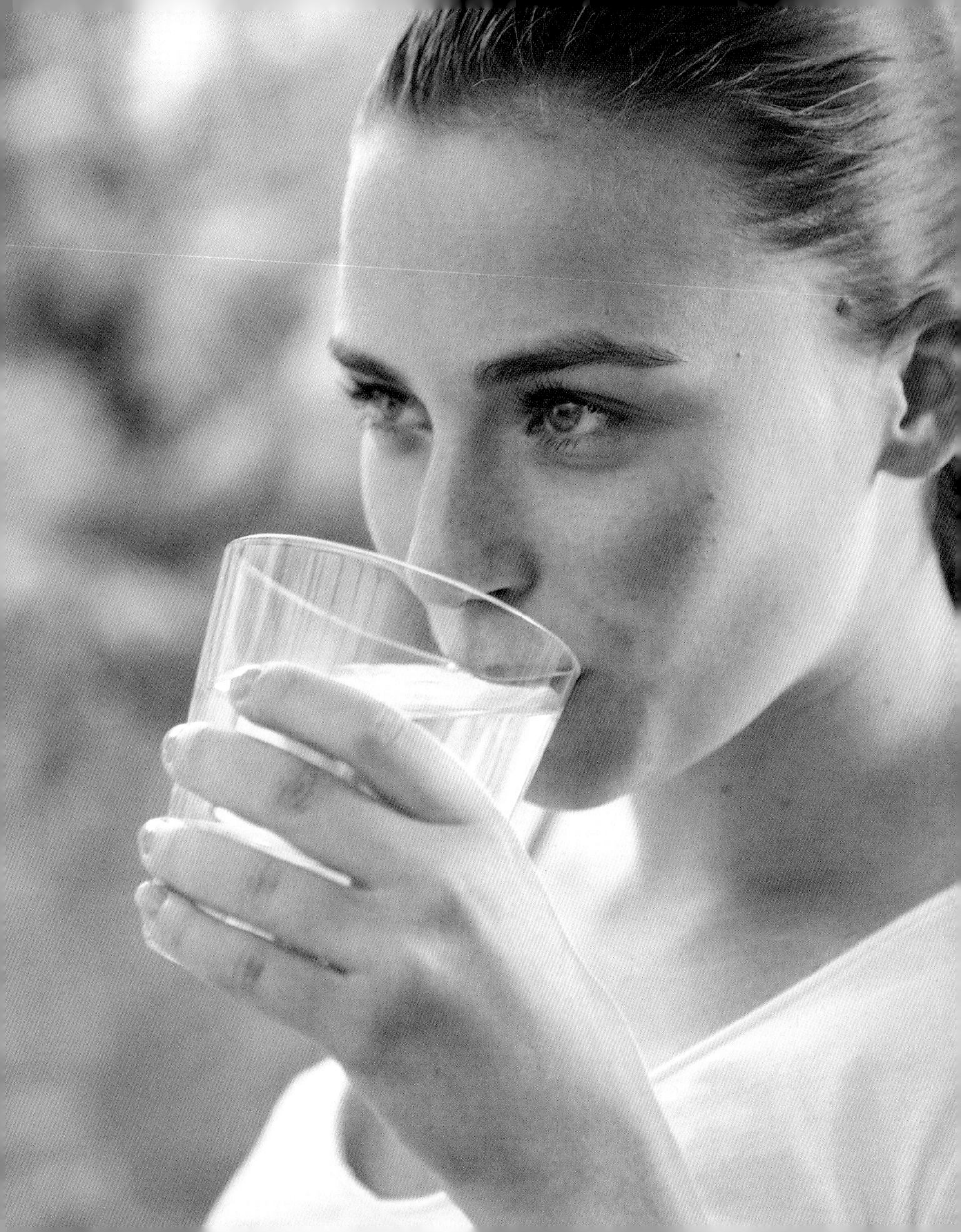

What emotionally affects this chakra?

Clairvoyants say this chakra naturally has an anticlockwise or feminine spin in both men and women. Psychologically it is linked to the Throat Chakra, which – if repressed – will have a detrimental knock-on effect. A healer will therefore often work upon both of these chakras in order to bring about balance.

In Eastern traditions this whole area is called the Hara, and is the centring point for body energies. In the Twelve Chakra System there is a separate Hara Chakra just above the Sacral.

The sacred dwelling place

Two 'serpents' of energy – the nadis called Ida and Pingala, representing dualities – bring energy up from the Base Chakra. They leave the Base where they were united and separate into male and female energies, then meet up once again in the Sacral Chakra in the 'sea of the Moon Goddess'. She symbolizes our sacred womb, the protectress of conception and development of new life. But in both sexes this chakra is also the sacred dwelling place of personal transformation, where we can move beyond the limitations of mind and emotions. When we are centred in this sacred place, we interact with our circumstances through mindfulness and generosity rather than through 'wants'. We can develop discernment, especially where sexuality is concerned, learn how to conserve energy, and what and whom we will allow to perceive our sacred centre.

However, if our own sexuality, mental stress or uncontrolled emotions are the issue, then this chakra requires balance, by looking closely at how we deal with duality in our lives. It requires us to centre an emotional and physical sense of self. Because ancestral and family issues are stored here, past-life regression will often move unhelpful blocks or lingering karmic ties.

On page 50 we explained how karma is closely linked to the Sacral Chakra and gave a modern definition of it. In

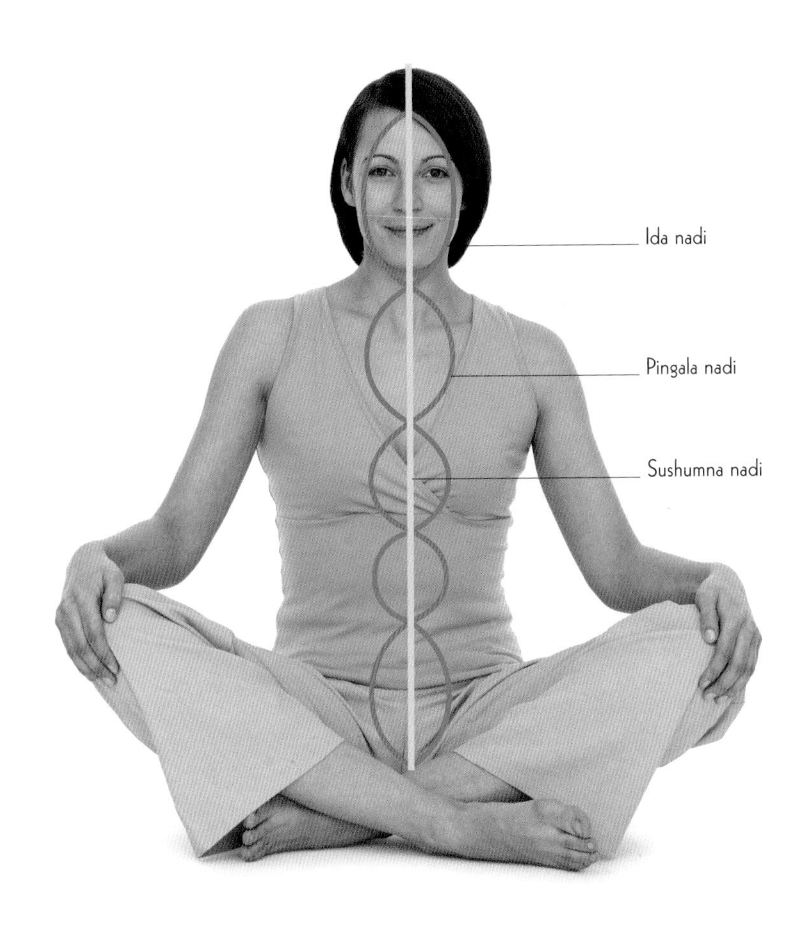

India, karma is considered to be the continual wheel of birth–death–rebirth, the cycle of cause and effect, or 'as ye sow, so shall ye reap'. Another thought-provoking definition is: 'Karma is an expression of the degree to which we have become separate from the Creator/God/Goddess.'

Balancing my Sacral Chakra

To help harmonize this important chakra you can regain equilibrium in a number of ways: through dance, laughter (a good 'belly' laugh), yoga, breathing exercises and visualization of orange-coloured light and even through eating orange-coloured food.

Free expression: dancing with light

As you will see in later chapters, a wonderful way to 'nourish' all your chakras is to feed them with beautiful harmonious music. To release your Sacral Chakra, and indeed balance all your chakras, dance! One evening choose to make a focus of a coloured candle, flowers and objects on a coloured cloth in the centre of a room. For the Sacral Chakra the colours should be predominantly orange, orange-yellow and orange-red. Then begin to play some joyful or perhaps passionate music. Stand very still, getting in touch with your inner energies. Breathe deeply, drawing in and around yourself the colour that you have chosen to work with.

Have a sense of your breath and of the music shifting colour to the place where it is most needed in your body. Begin to move that part of your body. Next, allow the music to flow into the rest of your body. Experience the exhilaration of spinning around, or the point of stillness as you hold a particular position. Be aware of how the music loosens your movements so that you use all the space in your room – lying and moving on the floor, or stretching toward the ceiling. Shiva, Lord of the Cosmic Dance, releases an ecstatic response within our chakras as we dance with joyous abandon.

The piece of music you have chosen will take you to the natural ending of your freely expressed Dance of Light. Lie down for a few minutes after you have finished. Your chakras, now harmonized, will make you feel refreshed and recharged.

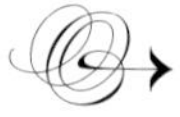

I'm not quite there yet Turn to Exercise 6: Sensing and Drawing my Sacral Chakra on page 66.

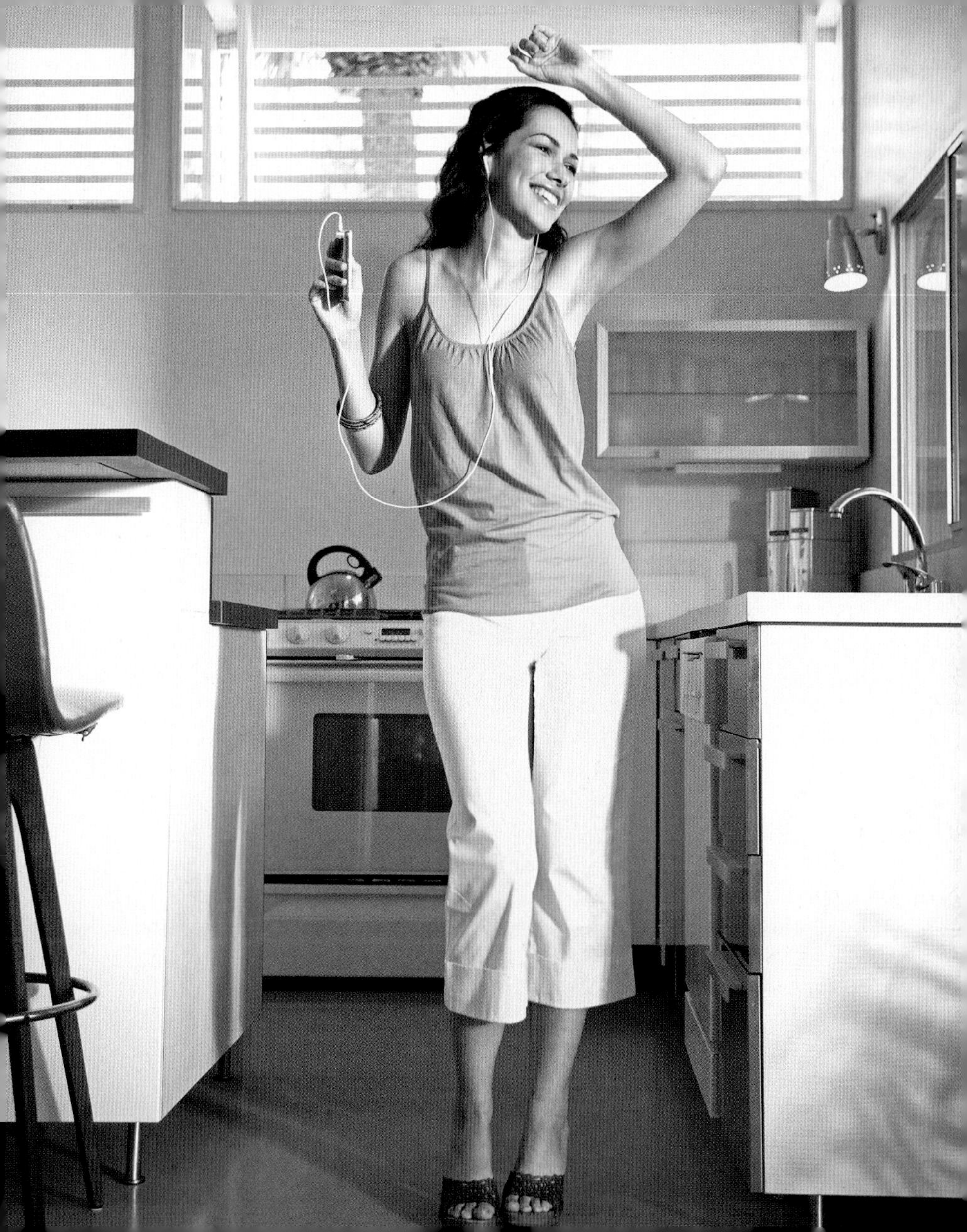

Using crystals to balance my chakras

By the time you have finished this book you may have made a collection of a number of crystals. If possible, this should include:

- Two 'grounding' stones (beach/river pebbles or obsidian)
- Two natural, clear quartz, pointed crystals, any size up to 10 cm (4 in) long
- A set of seven crystals: one in the colour of each major chakra; they may be small, inexpensive 'tumbled' (smooth and rounded) polished crystals
- You may also have a crystal pendulum. Keep your crystals in a special place, such as on your altar or sacred space, or wrap them carefully in red fabric – silk or natural fibre is best.

Cleanse your crystals before and after use. Cleansing methods include soaking the crystals in pure water; wafting them

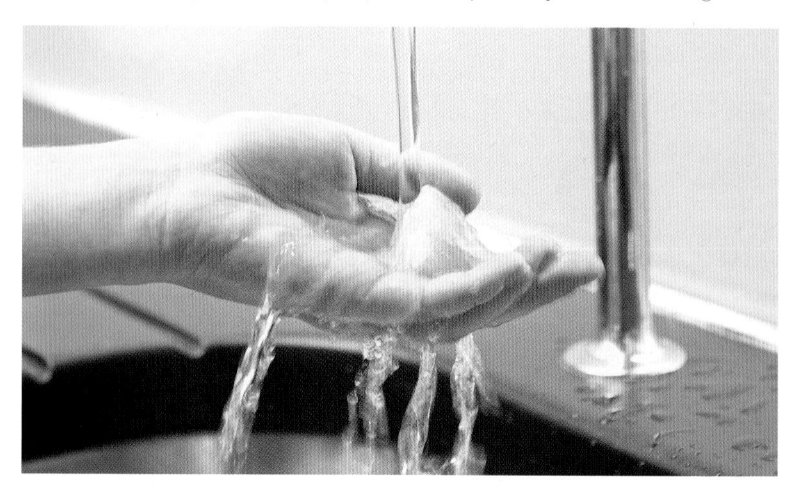

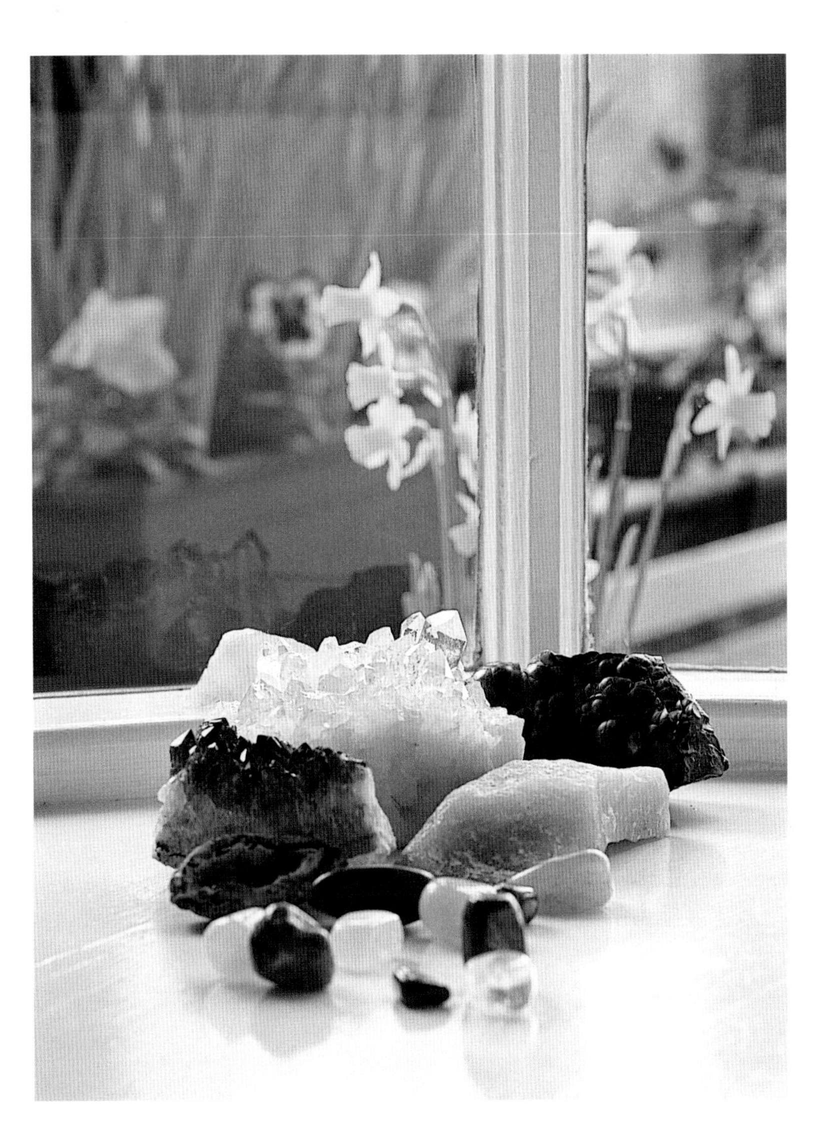

through incense smoke; prayer; flower remedies; or placing them on the earth or on a growing plant. You can also use the power of your mind: visualize them illuminated with clear white light. Occasionally you will need to recharge your crystals in sunlight or moonlight for 12 hours or so.

Before each exercise involving crystals, dedicate them to your chakra work, saying, for example, 'May this crystal draw upon the power of Unconditional Love and Light to balance my chakras and energies, for the highest good.'

Body/chakra boost

It has been proven that our physical and energy bodies respond to the presence of crystals. For this reason it is recommended that you obtain two pointed, clear quartz crystals, as mentioned above. Use the crystals to give a regular body/chakra boost and balance, to yourself or a friend, as follows.

First, find a pleasant place to lie down on your back, such as on a blanket in your sacred space. Then place one quartz crystal at the top of your head, pointing toward your feet, and the other crystal beyond your feet, pointing toward your head. *It is most important that the points of the quartz crystals point inward, because you wish to increase your subtle energy, not drain it away.*

Then just relax and let the crystals exert their influence. Finish by breathing deeply, stretching and sitting up slowly. Visualize the inner strength you could gain by making crystals a natural and intrinsic part of your life.

Work with your chakras now Turn to Exercise 9: Using Crystals on page 75, to begin to use crystals upon the Sacral Chakra.

SACRAL CHAKRA EXERCISES

The following exercises develop the Sacral Chakra or Svadisthana, which is your vitality centre. This chakra fulfils your life through appreciation of sexuality and creativity, and eventually will bring your feelings into a state of discernment. You will be using a pendulum to ascertain the chakra energies and how to rebalance them using various methods, such as Colour-Breathing a Rainbow (with the help of the CD) and crystals.

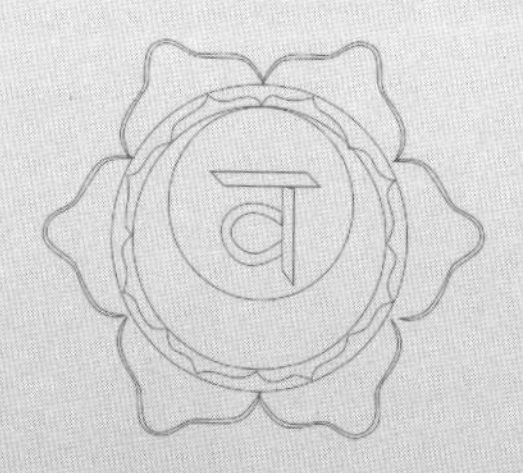

Developing intuition

Do this exercise before reading beyond this page. It will become a record of your Sacral Chakra – reflecting your emotions and your ability to trust others – to which you can refer back in order to chart your progress.

Exercise 6 SENSING AND DRAWING MY SACRAL CHAKRA

You will need: a set of coloured pencils or pens (all colours, including magenta); keep the book open, ready to colour in the body outline opposite, which represents *you* (sign and date it before you begin).

- **To begin,** take five minutes sitting in a quiet place, breathing slowly, relaxing and closing your eyes. Now start to sense your body and aura. Release any emotions that arise. Forget anything you have ever heard or read about chakras and auras. You are simply 'sensing' how your own unique energies are flowing at present. Check from your feet up to your head to pick up any little clues that your body is giving you. Sense your auric energy field around you as well. Now focus upon the Sacral Chakra area of your belly, navel and lower back. What is it 'telling' you? What can you sense? Does it feel free, flowing, harmonious? Or is an old pain or trauma held there? Does this area feel fluid and open, or have you shut off all feelings and thoughts of this chakra?
- **When you feel ready,** open your eyes and – immediately and without thinking – quickly colour in the Sacral Chakra area and any other parts of the body (and surrounding page) as you wish. There is no right or wrong place to apply the colour: it is entirely up to you.
- **Read the interpretation** on page 68 after completing this exercise.

My sensing and drawing my sacral chakra experience

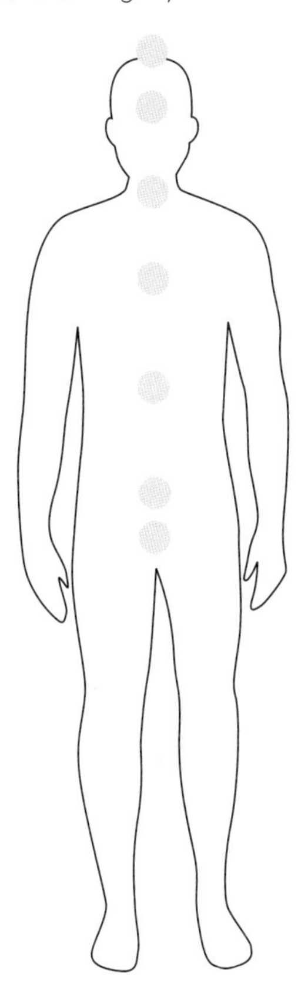

Date ______________________ Signature ______________________

Assessing my results for Exercise 6

A balanced Sacral Chakra will show strong and vibrant colours in the light-red/orange range. It will reflect your emotions and your ability to trust others. Like the Base Chakra, it is concerned with sexuality and life's pleasures, the basis of your vitality, your flexibility, security and love for yourself and all beings. Balance here indicates being joyful and able to take control of your own life – feeling happy in your own body.

An unbalanced Sacral Chakra will show either very weak or very strong colours. These colours may be dark shades – black, brown or grey. It will reflect addictions of all kinds, the inability to trust in the abundance of the universe, lack of vitality and sexual perversions and fears.

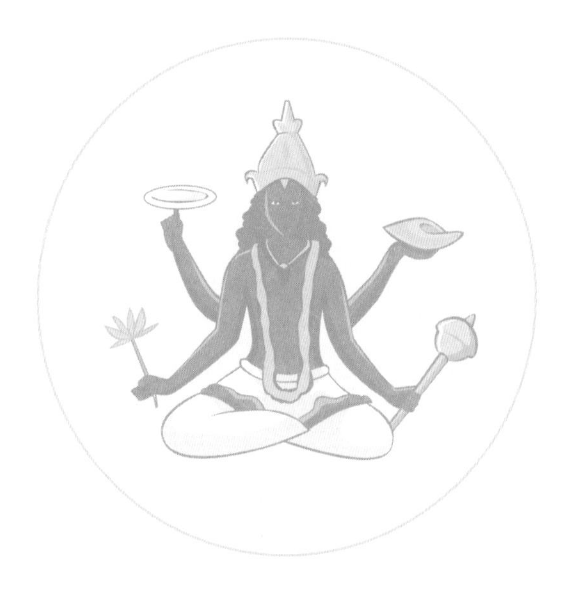

Scanning Sacral Chakra energy

Scanning is a method of using your hands to detect imbalances in the chakras and energy field. Your sensitivity gradually increases with practice. The minor chakras in the palms of your hands will pick up indications in different levels of the auric field, within the chakras and within the body itself. Eventually you will find this a very valuable 'diagnostic' method. Although at present you are using scanning on yourself, many healers who channel healing energy find it invaluable in their work.

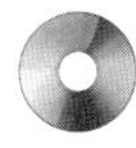

Exercise 7 SENSING MY SACRAL ENERGY

CD REFERENCE TRACK 2 (TO FOLLOW THE SCRIPT, TURN TO PAGE 110)

- **To begin,** ensure you will not be disturbed. Sit on your blanket and rub your hands vigorously together to stimulate pranic/ki energy to flow strongly through them. They should feel warm and energized. For this exercise you may use whichever hand you feel most comfortable with.
- **Lie down and relax,** using Track 2 on the CD, or following the instructions for Exercise 15: Complete Relaxation on page 110.
- **Keep your eyes closed** and begin to focus inwardly upon your Sacral Chakra energy. Increase that focus. After a few minutes move your hand slowly around the area of your Sacral Chakra, both within your auric field and on/over your body (this is 'scanning').
- **Notice whether your energy** feels different close into the body or further away. You may feel warmth/cold, lightness/heaviness, vibration/stillness, a colour, dense areas, vibrant areas or other sensations.

- **Remember what you feel,** so that you can record it on the following page.
- **To finish,** take a deep breath, stretch, roll onto one side of your body and sit up slowly.
- **Now consider** the questions on page 71.
- **Note:** You may use this exercise for sensing your Base, Solar Plexus, Heart, Throat, Third Eye and Crown Chakras as well.

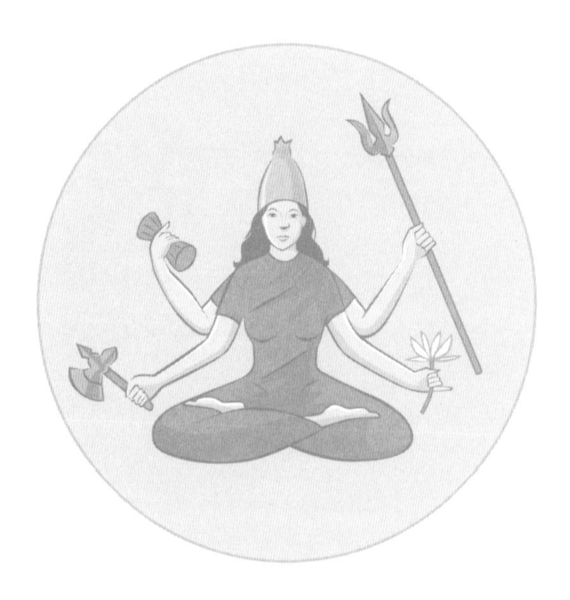

My sensing my Sacral energy experience

Date ______________________ Signature ______________________

This exercise was: Easy / Hard / Took a while to get used to it

What did I sense? (tick or expand on what you felt)

Heat ______________________ Cold ______________________

Lightness ______________________ Heaviness ______________________

Vibration ______________________ Stillness ______________________

A colour ______________________

Dense areas ______________________

Does this mean my Sacral Chakra energy is clogged/underactive? Yes / No

Do I need to activate it with colour-breathing orange? Yes / No
(if your answer is Yes, go to page 77)

Vibrant areas ______________________

Does this mean my Sacral Chakra energy is balanced? Yes / No

Did my Sacral Chakra energy seem overactive? Yes / No

Do I need to calm it with long, slow breaths of the colour peach? Yes / No
(if your answer is Yes, please do so)

Other sensations? Describe ______________________

Checking my Sacral Chakra is balanced

This dowsing exercise uses a pendulum to check whether your Sacral Chakra is balanced. As recommended on page 18, try to build up empathy and confidence in your pendulum, so that it can be used reliably to determine degrees of activity in each of your chakras.

Remember to avoid holding the pendulum over a chakra, particularly if it is a crystal one – instead, point a finger of the other hand toward and near the chakra in question. This ensures that the pendulum doesn't falsify the reading.

Below are just some of the questions you may ask. Or how about asking if you need aromatherapy or sound healing exercises? Perhaps you need yoga or other balancing body movements? Any questions that you ask must have only 'Yes' or 'No' answers.

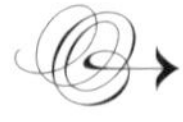

I'm not quite there yet Reread pages 18 and 19 for tips on how to use the pendulum.

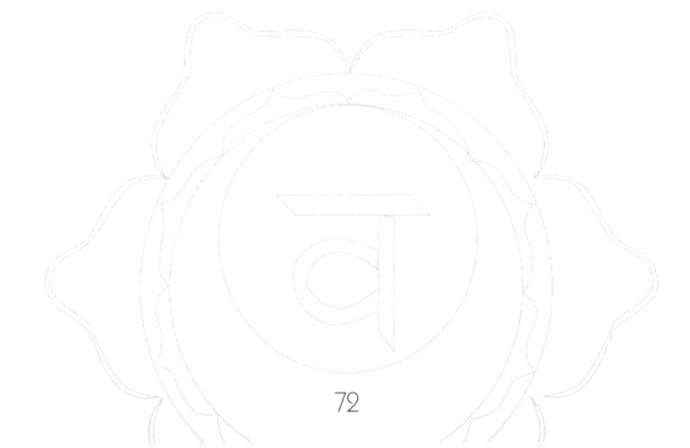

Exercise 8 DOWSING MY SACRAL CHAKRA

You will need: a pendulum, and a pen to record your results.

- **To begin,** remain focused and silent for a moment.
- **Then ask** the following questions:
  'Does this chakra require balancing?'
  'Is balance required on a physical level?'
  'Is balance required on a mental/emotional level?'
  'Is balance required on an energy level in my auric field?'

  It is also relevant to ask:
  'Is this chakra overactive or underactive?'
  'Is colour-breathing required?'
  'Is crystal balancing required?'
  'Is a change in my lifestyle required?'
- **Record your pendulum results** on page 74 (date and sign them), so that you can begin to see repeating (or varying) patterns of chakra activity. You may dowse just the Sacral Chakra, or you have space there to record the condition of all your chakras, if you wish. You can also compare the effects that various methods shown in this book have upon the chakras, by dowsing before and after any balancing work. It becomes very exciting when you do this, because you can start to see positive results.
- **As an optional method of dowsing,** use a blank 'body outline' (see pages 238–49). Sign it (this is your 'witness' or energy imprint). With the understanding that this body outline represents you, rest your index finger on each chakra in turn. Hold the pendulum in the other hand, well away from your physical body. Ask the questions given above. Record and date your results.

My dowsing my sacral chakra experience

Date ______________________ Signature ______________________

- Does this __________ Chakra require balancing? Yes / No
- Is balance required on a physical level? Yes / No
- Is balance required on a mental/emotional level? Yes / No
- Is balance required on an energy level in my auric field? Yes / No
- Is this __________ Chakra overactive? Yes / No
- Is colour-breathing required? Yes / No
- Is crystal balancing required? Yes / No
- Is a change in my lifestyle required? Yes / No
- Is this __________ Chakra underactive? Yes / No
- Is colour-breathing required? Yes / No
- Is crystal balancing required? Yes / No
- Is a change in my lifestyle required? Yes / No
- Ask any other questions that you wish to pose.

Circle the relevant states below:

Base Chakra	Balanced	Underactive	Overactive
Sacral Chakra	Balanced	Underactive	Overactive
Solar Plexus Chakra	Balanced	Underactive	Overactive
Heart Chakra	Balanced	Underactive	Overactive
Throat Chakra	Balanced	Underactive	Overactive
Third Eye Chakra	Balanced	Underactive	Overactive
Crown Chakra	Balanced	Underactive	Overactive

Clearing my aura

This exercise uses crystals to clear your aura and balance your Sacral Chakra. Depending on the effect that you require, you can use the following crystals:

- To balance: use moonstone or aquamarine
- To activate: use carnelian or fire opal
- To calm: use emerald, green aventurine or green calcite.

You can use this technique with the recommended crystals for each chakra, but work on just one chakra at a time.

Later, when you feel ready to do so, you may also work on the Sacral Chakra with any of the other balancing methods mentioned in this book. Consult the chart on page 51 to ascertain which aromatherapy oil to use, which yoga postures, colour breathing, and so on.

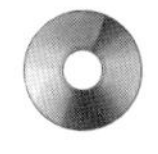

Exercise 9 USING CRYSTALS

CD REFERENCE TRACK 2 (TO FOLLOW THE SCRIPT, TURN TO PAGE 110)

- **Wear white clothes** or place a white sheet over your naked body. Lie down on a blanket and relax. Have your cleansed and dedicated crystal/s (see page 62) nearby.
- **When it feels right,** gently place your crystal over the Sacral Chakra. Then relax for ten minutes or so, before slowly coming back to everyday awareness. Now record your experience in the space provided on page 76.

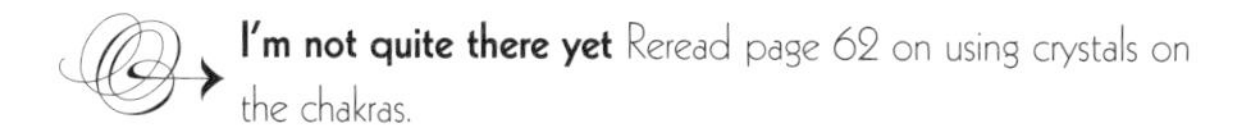

I'm not quite there yet Reread page 62 on using crystals on the chakras.

My using crystals experience

Date ______________________________

Chakra and crystal used ______________________________

What I wanted to achieve ______________________________

What I felt ______________________________

____

What I would like to do next time I try this exercise ______________________________

____

Does my chakra feel balanced? ______________________________

If not, ask the chakra what it needs. Close your eyes and talk to your chakra.

Record here what it needs ______________________________

____

Record here what you have done as a result, and the date ______________________________

____

____

____

Breathing colour into all the chakras

This exercise helps you to breathe colour into all of your seven chakras, in a continuation of the relaxation exercise on page 110.

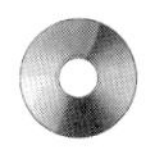

Exercise 10 COLOUR-BREATHING A RAINBOW

CD REFERENCE TRACK 2 (OPTIONAL) (TO FOLLOW THE SCRIPT, TURN TO PAGE 110) **CD REFERENCE** TRACK 1 (TO FOLLOW THE SCRIPT, SEE BELOW)

- **To begin**, lie flat on your back with your feet slightly apart. If you have a back problem, bend your knees, but keep your feet flat and about 75 cm (30 in) apart and support your knees with cushions. Close your eyes. Take three deep breaths, and breathe out any feelings of stress when you exhale. Check through your body from your feet to the top of your head to ensure you are relaxed.
- **Focus on your Base Chakra** and legs. Visualize your incoming breath as a bright-red light. 'Pull' and direct it to your Base.
- **Focus on your Sacral Chakra** and abdomen. Visualize your incoming breath as a vibrant orange light. 'Pull' and direct it to your Sacrum.
- **Focus on your Solar Plexus Chakra,** stomach and digestive organs. Visualize your incoming breath as a sunny yellow light. 'Pull' and direct it to your Solar Plexus.
- **Focus on your Heart Chakra** and chest. Visualize your incoming breath as a bright grass-green light. 'Pull' and direct it to your Heart.
- **Focus on your Throat Chakra,** neck, throat, face and back of head. Visualize your incoming breath as a bright turquoise-blue light. 'Pull' and direct it to your Throat.

- **Focus on your Third Eye Chakra,** the centre of your brow, eyes and brain. Visualize your incoming breath as a clear deep-blue light. 'Pull' and direct it to your Third Eye.
- **Focus on your Crown Chakra,** the top of your head and just above your head. Visualize your incoming breath as a clear violet light. 'Pull' and direct it to your Crown.
- **Now visualize clear golden-white light** streaming into the top of your head. Pull the golden-white light into each chakra in turn: Crown, Third Eye, Throat, Heart, Solar Plexus, Sacral, Base. Take the golden-white light right down to your feet, and release it through your soles into the Earth and the Earth Star Chakra beneath you.
- **Return to a normal breathing pattern** and enjoy the feeling of your recharged chakras. Wait a few moments, then stretch and slowly sit up.
- **Now consider** the questions on the opposite page.

My colour-breathing a rainbow experience

Date ______________________________

Is it becoming easier to do colour-breathing? Yes / No / A bit / Don't know

Base Chakra/red breath
How did my chakra feel? ______________________________
Did it change my mood? ______________________________
Did it bring up a particular emotion or thought? ______________________________
Does my Base Chakra now feel balanced? ______________________________

Sacral Chakra/orange breath
How did my chakra feel? ______________________________
Did it change my mood? ______________________________
Did it bring up a particular emotion or thought? ______________________________
Does my Sacral Chakra now feel balanced? ______________________________

Solar Plexus Chakra/yellow breath
How did my chakra feel? ______________________________
Did it change my mood? ______________________________
Did it bring up a particular emotion or thought? ______________________________
Does my Solar Plexus Chakra now feel balanced? ______________________________

Heart Chakra/grass-green breath
How did my chakra feel? ______________________________
Did it change my mood? ______________________________
Did it bring up a particular emotion or thought? ______________________________
Does my Heart Chakra now feel balanced? ______________________________

Throat Chakra/turquoise-blue breath
How did my chakra feel? ______________________________
Did it change my mood? ______________________________
Did it bring up a particular emotion or thought? ____________________
Does my Throat Chakra now feel balanced? ____________________

Third Eye Chakra/clear deep-blue breath
How did my chakra feel? ______________________________
Did it change my mood? ______________________________
Did it bring up a particular emotion or thought? ____________________
Does my Third Eye Chakra now feel balanced? ____________________

Crown Chakra/violet breath
How did my chakra feel? ______________________________
Did it change my mood? ______________________________
Did it bring up a particular emotion or thought? ____________________
Does my Base Chakra now feel balanced? ____________________

Next time I do this exercise, should I allow myself more time? ____________

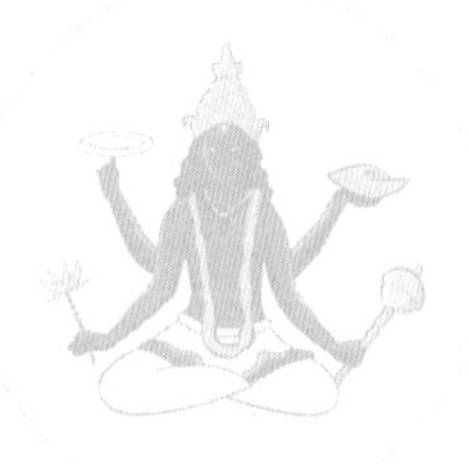

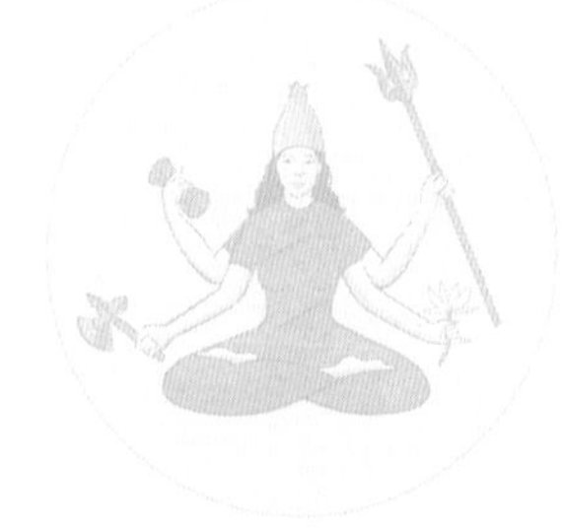

THE SOLAR PLEXUS CHAKRA: MANIPURA

Work with your chakras now Before you read further, turn to Exercise 11: Sensing and Drawing my Solar Plexus Chakra on page 98.

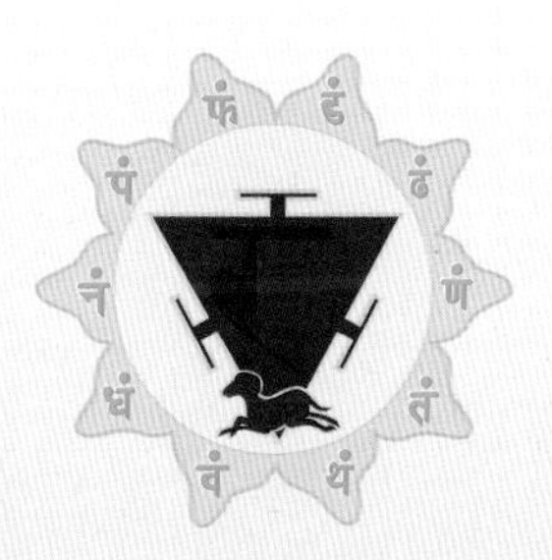

About my Solar Plexus Chakra

Keypoints: Resonates with the Fire element and the colour yellow/gold; concerned with power, empowerment by overcoming our limiting personal ego, becoming non-judgmental and finding our own truth.

The third chakra, the Solar Plexus, is our power base – flexibility here allows us to break away from external control. The Sanskrit name, *Manipura*, means 'the place of jewels', indicating that it is a precious powerful link to our body.

The element of Fire rules the active 'solar power station' of this chakra, and the sun's bio-compatible energies, charged with *prana*, are stored here. In Western esoteric teachings, salamander Fire elementals are interdimensional beings who control, live in and direct the energy of fire. They are keepers of sacred flames. Understanding them aids your appreciation of diverse subtle energies and the secret workings of this chakra.

The seat of the emotions lies within the Solar Plexus Chakra. The more our inappropriate emotions are processed through it, the more the Fire energy there will burn them up. *The ego is closely allied to this chakra* – it is a modern trend to refer persistently to the ego, a psychological construct not recognized until the 20th century. In the past the Devil sat on our shoulder, but now it is our ego that needs to be put in the fire of transformation. Some people consider that ego becomes apparent in childhood due to demands to conform and succeed. If so, then ego is an addiction every bit as powerful as smoking or drinking. Are you using your ego as an excuse? Reflect that you are now an adult, working consciously upon your chakra system to evolve yourself. Every ego eventually has to be released, if humanity is to reach Oneness and Unity.

Golden-yellow light stimulates this chakra. At auric-field level the Solar Plexus Chakra is linked to the secondary minor chakras of the stomach and liver and two minor spleen chakras.

CHART OF THE SOLAR PLEXUS CHAKRA

Colour of influence	Yellow
Complementary light colour	Violet
Colour to calm	Violet
Physical location	Between bottom of sternum and navel
Physiological system	Metabolic/digestive
Endocrine system	Islets of Langerhans (groups of cells in the pancreas)
Key issues	Power, fear, anxiety and introversion
Inner teaching	Honouring the wisdom of others, leading to personal empowerment
Energy action	Transduces incoming solar and *pranic* energy; expels negative body energies
Balancing crystals	Citrine quartz
Balancing aromatherapy oils	Clary sage, juniper, geranium
Balancing herbal teas	Juniper/fennel or detox tea; or a soothing mix of chamomile, marshmallow root, raspberry leaf, fenugreek seed, meadowsweet, slippery elm bark, comfrey and liquorice root
Balancing yoga position (*asana*)	Gomukasana (cow), Ardha matsyendrasana I (sitting spinal twist), Ustrasana (camel)
Mantra/tone	RAM in note of E (sounding like 'rarm')
Helpful musical instruments/music	Loud brass/saxophone to clear 'dead' energy, classical guitar music to calm
Planet/astrological sign/natural House	Sun/Moon/Leo/Cancer/fifth: Love/fourth: Family
Reiki hand position	Lying on back: both palms over the Solar Plexus and stomach; lying on front: both palms on middle back/lungs
Power animal (Native American tradition)	Birds and especially eagles

Body/Solar Plexus connections

The action of the Solar Plexus Chakra on the glandular system occurs through the pancreas, which has small clumps of cells (called the islets of Langerhans), the source of insulin, which is involved in the metabolism of sugar. The physical location of the chakra stretches from the bottom of the breastbone (sternum) to the navel, covering a large area, including the stomach, gall bladder and liver – organs primarily concerned with the digestive system. The coeliac plexus is a network of nerves that meet here. Additionally, the sympathetic nervous system and the health of our muscles are influenced by this chakra.

Links with diabetes and cancer

In the case of diabetes, a holistic practitioner may work with a client to establish why they do not enable sweetness (both of sugars and of personality) to be properly absorbed. From a body/mind perspective, sweetness or love in our lives can become unbalanced. Often love is overprotective or smothering (as from mother to child), and so repetitive patterns of diabetes frequently occur in families. Regular whole-body chakra balancing is required as well as medical treatment.

In cancer and pre-cancerous indications, this chakra can be holding onto unprocessed emotions of anger, fear or hate. Genetic analysis of tumours by the Howard Hughes Medical Institute and Johns Hopkins University in the USA (reported in 2010) suggested that the first cellular mutations may occur 20 years before they develop and become fatal.

Balancing the Solar Plexus may influence your level of wellness. Its natural function is to process energies both from the lower chakras and from the Heart Chakra. Balance may be achieved through healing, meditation, visualization, colour-breathing, using crystals (particularly green emerald or citrine quartz) or simply by consciously breathing in the power of the sun. While these modalities do not replace medical treatment, they do enhance and support medical techniques, through the body's innate desire to return to equilibrium and sustain its own healing, without dependency.

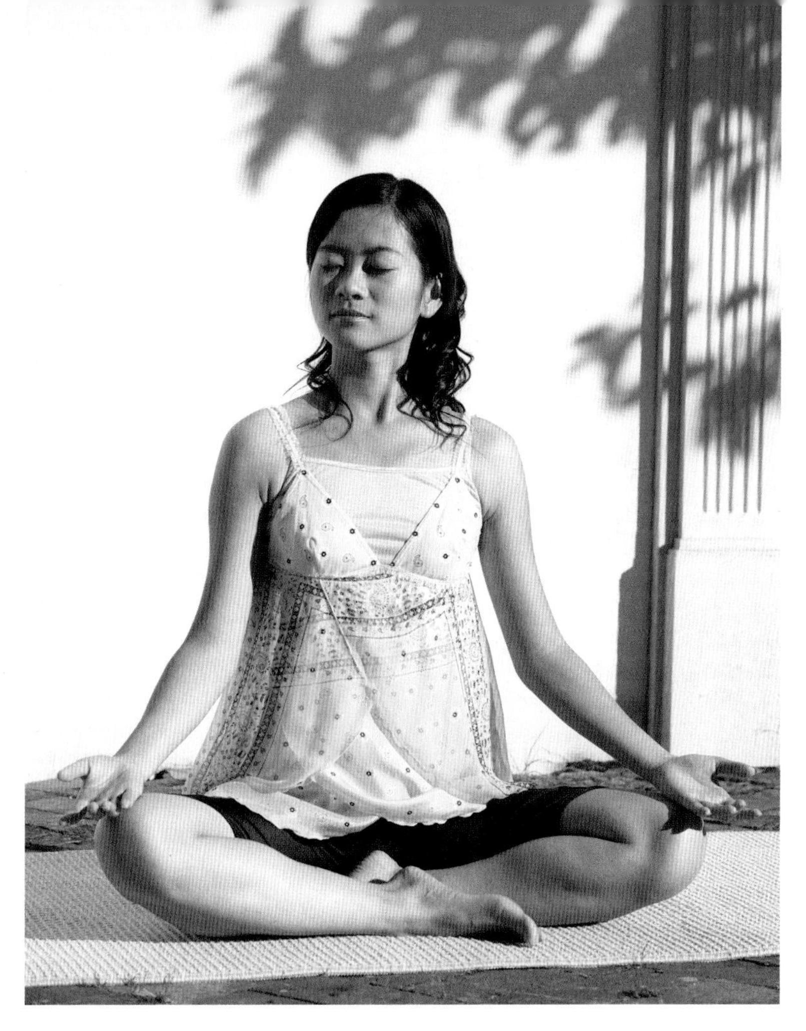

Work with your chakras now Turn to Exercise 12: Sensing my Solar Plexus Energy on page 101, to further develop your intuition.

Optional advanced exercises See pages 174, 197, 199 and 206 for more advanced work.

The energy of this chakra

This chakra is where upward-flowing Earth energy meets downward-flowing energy called apana – a specialized type of *prana*.

The expression 'To have a gut feeling' – meaning a sense of feeling something at a very deep level – is actually the Solar Plexus Chakra in action. It enables us to discriminate between good and bad feelings. Maybe you have felt 'butterflies in your stomach' – or a tightening of the whole area – just before an important event. This is the chakra closing down a little, becoming more passive, and pulling in and slightly away from the physical body as a form of protection.

The main action of energy entering the Solar Plexus Chakra assists transmutation and the assimilation of food into a type of coloured light/*pranic* energy that body cells can use. This is why we say it is concerned not only with emotions, but with digestive processes and with nourishing our bodies. One way to harmonize this chakra is by increasing intake of yellow-coloured food, remembering the cleansing properties of lemons, for instance, and the soothing properties of bananas. Other ways are shown on the following pages.

The Solar Plexus is like an inner fire of transmutation, burning up negativity and harmonizing your emotions. If you are going through a period of inner turbulence, allocate some 'me' time. Do something you enjoy and try to relax. Then sit quietly and look at the situation in which you find yourself or which you have drawn toward yourself as a life lesson. Remember that, at soul level, we learn from seemingly the most dire situations and gain inner strength as a result.

Settle down and, as you breathe in, take back all the judgments you have made. Hold them with your breath. Then, as you breathe out, release them one by one. Make sure they have all gone. Maybe you need to expel them with a great sigh. Finally, accept the situation as it is. Be gentle with yourself and with those around you. Perhaps you would like to sit with your partner, or with a friend who is willing to help you, and do the exercises together?

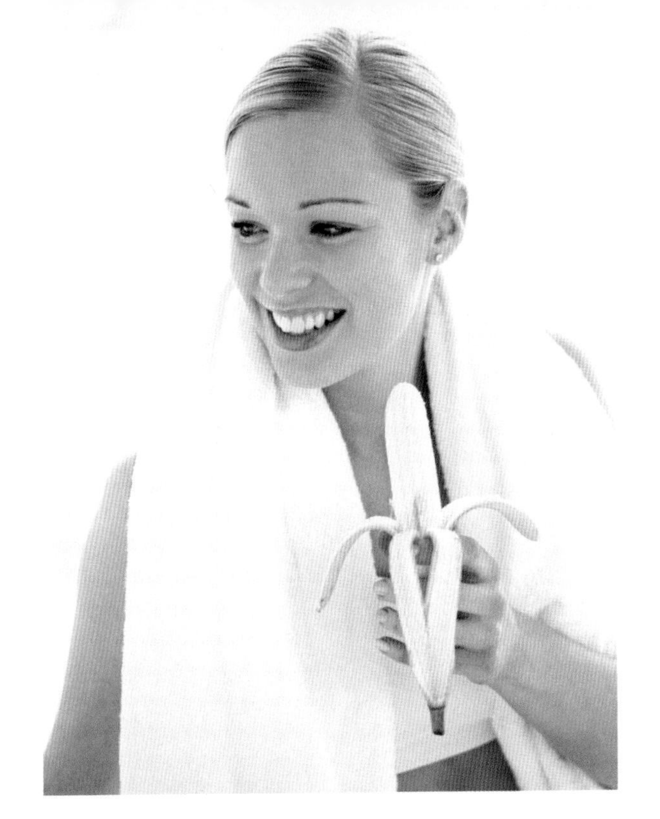

Work with your chakras now Turn to Exercise 13: Dowsing my Solar Plexus Chakra on page 103, to check the balance of this chakra. You can do this both before and after doing any 'remedial' exercises or inner work upon yourself. Remember that it is useful to record your results.

Optional advanced exercise Alternatively, turn to Exercise 28: Releasing Negative Patterns on page 199, for more advanced work, and read page 216.

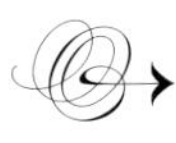

I'm not quite there yet Go back to Exercise 10: Colour-Breathing a Rainbow on page 77 and CD reference Track 1.

What influences this chakra?

The region of the Solar Plexus Chakra is known in Traditional Chinese Medicine as 'the Triple Warmer' because of the heat generated there during digestion. When this heat is properly regulated through a wholesome and balanced diet, we have health and wellness. However, the nutritive value of junk food and fast food is insufficient to maintain health at many levels. Not only does our body

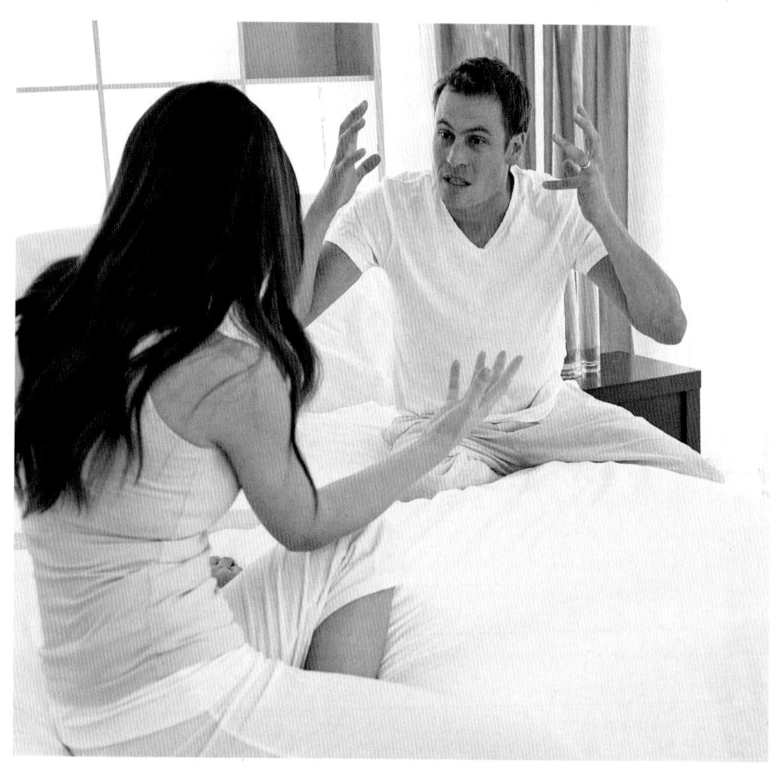

suffer on this type of diet, but our energy reserves also become depleted. If this applies to you, endeavour to correct your diet while simultaneously undertaking the exercises in this book.

Body/mind connections

Sometimes the physical Solar Plexus is referred to as our 'lower mind', because the nerve ganglion there is considered to be a kind of 'visceral brain' where our digestive processes are regulated. Hence this area is subject to various stress-related disorders, such as ulcers. On a body/mind level, people suffering from ulcers may live too much in their mind and be emotionally repressed.

Energy blockages at the Solar Plexus can manifest as domination, anger and abuse. A person exhibiting these qualities of internal conflict becomes stuck at this level, between dominance and submission, where the only escape seems to be aggression or timidity respectively. These body/mind symptoms finally manifest as adrenal-gland weakness, leading to loss of energy and lack of vitality. When considering body/mind connections, do realize that they are often deeply buried in the subconscious and, while it is acceptable to work upon them yourself, it can be damaging to use them as an excuse or as a 'diagnosis' on other people. Most of the inner conflicts or spiritual-growth opportunities within the chakras are not usually recognized consciously, and it would be hurtful to express them about others unless you are in a therapist–client role.

However, this book is about healing yourself, and *the Solar Plexus is a vital chakra centre to take care of*, because a whole range of emotions can cause it to be overstimulated. Through my energy work I have noticed that misuse of personal power is a result of overactivity of the Solar Plexus, while introversion of personality is a result of underactivity. The happy balance is personal empowerment that honours the wisdom and knowledge of others.

Work with your chakras now Turn to Exercise 14 Breathing in Solar Energies on page 107, for an excellent way to learn how to balance the Solar Plexus Chakra.

Calming my emotions

Has your Solar Plexus Chakra gone into emotional overload? Are you stressed? Does your whole Solar Plexus area feel 'knotted up', or tight and painful, if you prod it with your fingers? This can indicate long-held stress or the kind of tension that builds up before a particularly important event, such as speaking in public.

Firm circular massage in a clockwise direction will usually give relief, using aromatherapy oils such as chamomile to calm the area. You could also try geranium essential oil, because it helps to regulate hormone secretion throughout the whole endocrine system. Also helpful will be a soak in a warm bath containing a few drops of pure chamomile or clary sage essential oil, followed by a cool shower. This releases negativity into the water, leaving you feeling refreshed.

Using a Yantra

In the Indian tradition a Yantra – which means a mapping 'machine' of sacred design in Sanskrit – takes you into a space of relaxation. The Shri Yantra is a traditional design formed by nine interlocking triangles, which surround and radiate out from the central bindu (dot) point, the junction between the physical universe and its unmanifest source. Four of the triangles point upward, representing the Divine Masculine Shiva, and the other five point downward, representing the Divine Feminine Shakti – and hence their union. Together the nine triangles are interlaced to form 43 smaller triangles in a weblike structure that is symbolic of the entire cosmos, or a womb of Creation through the union of Shiva and Shakti.

You may use a Yantra as a focus to still your mind. Look gently at the centre of the Shri Yantra opposite, trying not to blink or close your eyes for some minutes. After a while close your eyes, but keep the image in your 'mind's eye'. Next open your eyes, expanding your focus from the centre of the Shri Yantra to the whole image. Do this repeatedly, looking back at the Yantra when you need to, until your mind is still. This practice reduces stress and develops concentration, leading to relaxation and meditation and eventually to enlightenment.

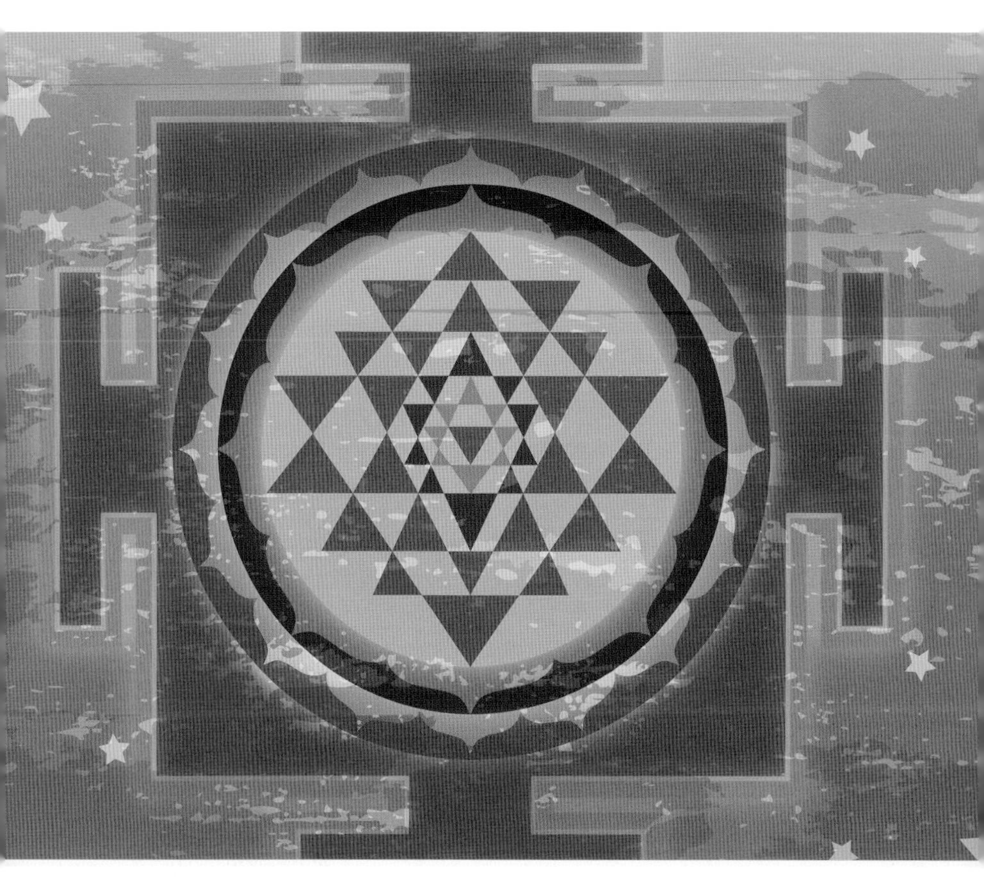

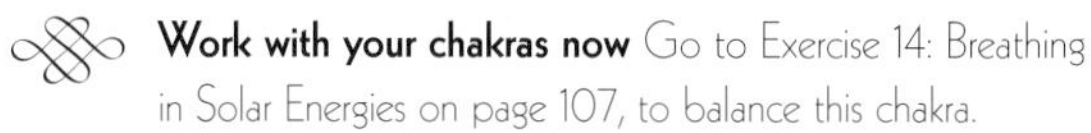

Work with your chakras now Go to Exercise 14: Breathing in Solar Energies on page 107, to balance this chakra.

I'm not quite there yet Read pages 92–3 to learn how to balance the Solar Plexus Chakra. Then consider treating yourself to a wonderfully relaxing aromatherapy bath.

Balancing my Solar Plexus Chakra

Relaxation techniques and yoga are both good ways of balancing the Solar Plexus Chakra. 'Your Health is in your own Hands', so make a start on healing yourself using self-taught practices now.

Yoga

You are strongly recommended to take up regular practice of an energy-based discipline that harmonizes the Solar Plexus and all the chakras – t'ai chi ch'uan or yoga are ideal. The development and function of our chakras are of primary importance in yogic tradition, and present-day knowledge of the chakras can be traced to some of the most ancient written texts in the world. These include the *Hathapradipika*, the *Yoga Sutras of Patanjali* and the *Bhagavad Gita*.

For thousands of years Indian mystics knew the nature of chakra energies, and Ayurvedic doctors (traditional healers who restored balance through the 'doshas' or elements of yoga teachings) practised a holistic approach to healthcare. Then at the end of the 19th century meditation arrived in Western esoteric circles. It was like a lotus plant that had lain dormant in Western consciousness. Later many kinds of meditation developed and suddenly blossomed during the late 20th century into a beautiful flower.

Also arising in the East was Shaktism, an organized religious sect dating from the 5th century, and it is their interpretation of the chakras that is most widely used today. In the charts accompanying each of the seven chakras you will find some recommended yoga *asanas* (postures), and there is considerably more about yoga in *The Chakra Bible*.

Relaxation techniques

Stress and tension are necessary for success; but when they become prolonged, or our reaction to them is inappropriate, the body protests in various ways, leading eventually to illness. However, your body has a remarkable ability to heal itself, if you give it the

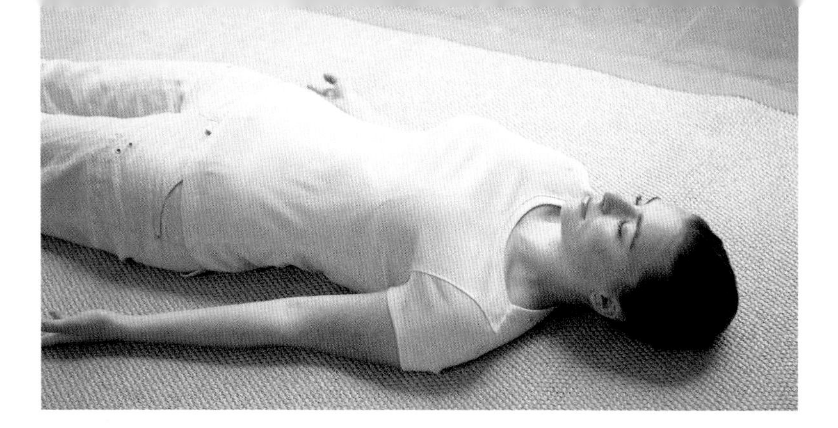

chance. To counter stress, you will find a tried-and-tested relaxation technique on page 110. A technique such as this can be learned by anyone and can then be applied to situations in daily life. It involves no drugs and there are only *pleasant* side-effects. You are asked to participate fully and to practise using the CD supplied with this book. As you begin to lower your stress levels, regular deep relaxation will prove its worth.

During relaxation you remain awake, although afterwards you may feel as if you have had a long, refreshing sleep. When you first learn the technique you will be focusing intently on every part of your body. It is known that whenever you do this, your energy body, chakras and aura receive beneficial activation. Medical science also demonstrates that if you think about a particular part of your physical body, blood flow there increases and healing can occur more rapidly.

With deep relaxation you:

- Learn how to breathe fully and have a positive attitude to life
- Naturally bring your chakra energies into balance
- Can expect to improve your physical skills and performance
- Are likely to enrich your personal relationships, because it is easier to get on with people when you are relaxed
- Can change your habits, sleep better, feel more fulfilled and perhaps will not need to combat your stress using cigarettes, drink or drugs.

Work with your chakras now Turn to Exercise 13: Dowsing my Solar Plexus Chakra on page 103, to check whether this chakra is balanced.

Aromatherapy for my chakras

In the evolutionary plan that includes all life on this planet, flowers are the essence and ultimate concentration of a plant's life-force, which is a specialized type of *pranic* energy. They end the cycle of plant growth by providing fertility mechanisms for the reproduction of the species.

Pure essential oils are processed from all parts of plants using different methods, such as steam distillation or maceration. Flowers provide the most fragrant and beneficial oils for the chakras; for example, rose, lavender, linden, ylang-ylang, jasmine, chamomile and neroli. This is because the vibrational level of a flower essential oil is highly charged and compatible with spiritual, mental and emotional dimensions of the human body through a process of resonance. Leaves and the woody parts of aromatic herbs are used to provide slightly larger, less expensive quantities of essential oil; for example, sage, juniper, rosemary, thyme and basil.

These oils, while still working upon the chakra system, offer measurable benefits to the physical body, improving the function of all systems, from relaxing the muscles to balancing hormones. All essential oils are volatile by nature and their small molecular structure easily permeates the skin or is inhaled. Once inside the body, minute aromatized particles circulate through the bloodstream, bringing therapeutic effects to specific organs and body systems. The essential oil that you choose can therefore produce a therapeutic, relaxing, stimulating or sensual effect.

There are many different ways of using essential oils, including the following:

- **Oil diffusers**, sometimes called vaporizers or oil burners (although you should never burn precious essential oil!) give a wonderful boost to the emotions and help respiratory conditions. Simply place a little water in the diffuser's reservoir, add up to five drops of pure essential oil and light a 'tea light' candle underneath.
- **Aromatherapy massage** uses essential oils diluted with a base 'carrier' oil, such as sweet almond, grapeseed or

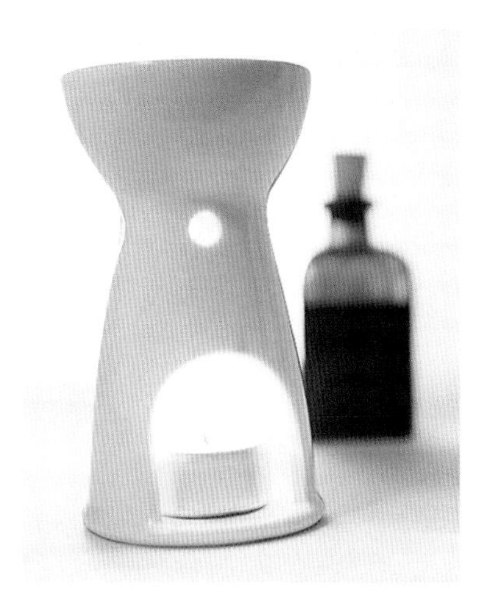

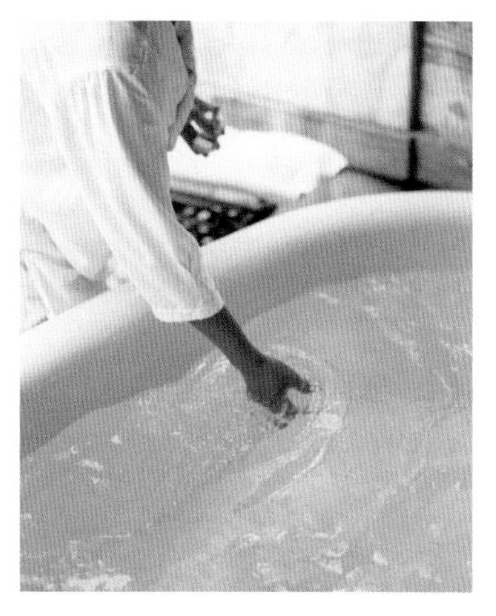

avocado. The dilution rate for adults is: 2.5 per cent essential oil to 97.5 per cent base/carrier oil. To ascertain the correct level, measure your base oil in millilitres and divide by two; the answer gives the number of drops of essential oil required. For example, 20 ml of base oil requires a maximum of ten drops. It is far better to mix your own oil when needed than buy ready-made preparations, because you can assure yourself of the quality of the oils. If you cannot afford a professional massage, ask a friend or treat yourself by massaging the oil into any appropriate parts of your body that you can reach, using firm circular movements.

- **Aromatherapy bathing** is a luxurious way to pamper yourself. Run a warm bath and, just before you get in, add no more than ten drops of your chosen essential oil in the base oil or even in milk. Relax and rebalance your whole chakra system.
- **Steam inhalation** helps the respiratory system. It is excellent for coughs, colds, sore throats and sinus infections – all of which indicate that your Throat, Heart and Thymus Chakras are under stress. Boil 1 litre (1 3/4 pt) of water and pour it into a bowl. Add ten drops of essential oil or a big bunch of a fresh herb (rosemary or thyme are excellent). Put a towel over your head and inhale the vapour for a

few minutes at a time until the water has cooled.

- **Room-spray fragrance** is excellent for cleansing crystals before and after use, as well as for scenting and cleansing your sacred space. Take a glass spray bottle and for each 5 ml of water use up to three drops of essential oil. For example, a 100 ml bottle will take 60 drops of essential oil. Add 10 ml of alcohol (such as vodka) to disperse it.
- **Purification breathing** uses essential oils to assist the release of despair, depression and other negative states of mind. Use an uplifting oil such as juniper, myrrh, basil or frankincense in an oil diffuser/vaporizer and go into a deep-breathing exercise and colour-breathing visualization for your chosen chakra. Continue until you feel purified and as if your mind is clear. Finally, take a breath of pure white light to recharge your entire body and subtle-energy system.
- **Anointing the chakra area** with essential oil diluted with a carrier oil.
- **Ceremonial cleansing of the auric field** or 'aura brushing', by spraying your auric field (avoid the eyes) to disperse any heavy vibrations trapped there. Use a mix of water, oil and alcohol, as recommended for room sprays.
- **Note:** Never take essential oils orally. Test them first, if your skin is likely to be sensitive. Do not use essential oils at all during pregnancy or on children under the age of 12, except under the supervision of a professional. Some oils, such as clary sage and chamomile, should not be used if you need to drive a car afterwards, for they make you too relaxed.

Seven useful essential oils for the chakras

You will find a number of recommended essential oils for the chakras in the charts that accompany the opening of each chapter, of which the best are:

- Base Chakra – Patchouli
- Sacral Chakra – Sandalwood
- Solar Plexus Chakra – Juniper
- Heart Chakra – Rose
- Throat Chakra – Lavender
- Brow Chakra – Frankincense
- Crown Chakra – Ylang-ylang

SOLAR PLEXUS CHAKRA EXERCISES

The following exercises develop the Solar Plexus Chakra or Manipura, the 'power-centre', where solar energies from food are transformed into light 'nutrients' for your body. You will be shown ways to increase solar light in your energy field, as well as continuing 'colour-breathing', 'scanning', dowsing with a pendulum and relaxing completely with the help of the CD.

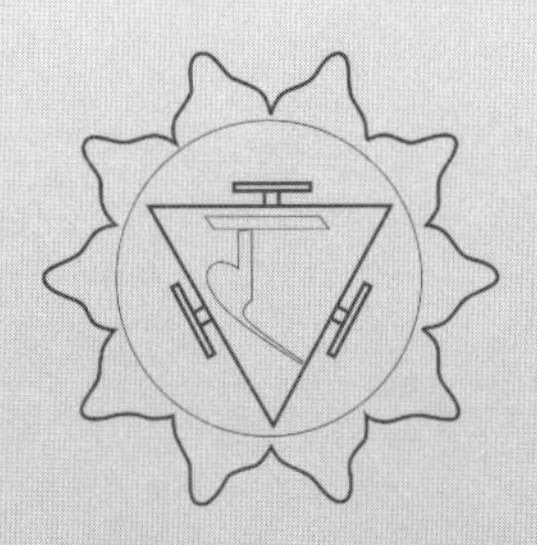

Developing intuition

Do this exercise before reading beyond this page. It will become a record of your Solar Plexus Chakra – showing how much you respect yourself and others and how accurate your 'gut feelings' are – to which you can refer back to chart your progress.

Exercise 11 SENSING AND DRAWING MY SOLAR PLEXUS CHAKRA

You will need: a set of coloured pencils or pens (all colours, including magenta); keep the book open, ready to colour in the body outline opposite, which represents you (sign and date it before you begin).

- **To begin,** take five minutes sitting in a quiet place, breathing slowly, relaxing and closing your eyes. Now start to sense your body and your aura. Release any emotions that arise. Forget anything you have ever heard or read about chakras and auras. You are simply 'sensing' how your own unique energies are flowing at present. Check from your feet up to your head to pick up any little clues that your body is giving you. Sense your auric energy field around you as well. Now focus upon your Solar Plexus Chakra area, which is centred slightly below the ribs. What is it 'telling' you? What can you sense? Does it feel free, flowing, harmonious? Or is an old pain or trauma held there? Does this area feel fluid and open – or have you shut off all feelings and thoughts of this chakra?
- **When you feel ready,** open your eyes and – immediately and without thinking – quickly colour in the Base Chakra area and any other parts of the body (and the surrounding page) as you wish. There is no right or wrong place to apply the colour: it is entirely up to you.
- **Read the interpretation** on page 100 after completing this exercise.

My sensing and drawing my solar plexus chakra experience

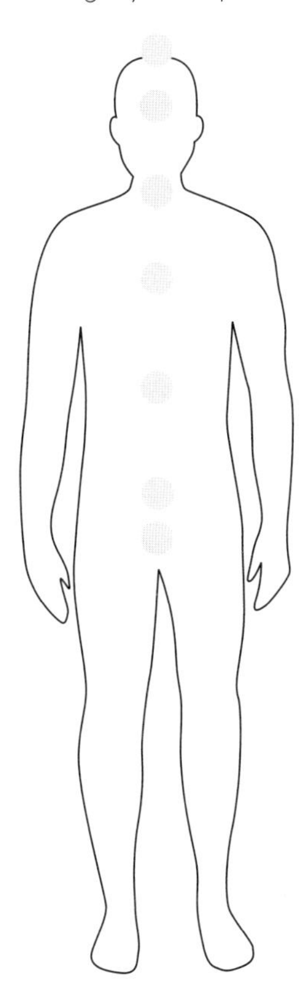

Date ______________________ Signature ______________________

Assessing my results for Exercise 11

A balanced Solar Plexus Chakra will show strong and vibrant colours in the light-orange/yellow range. It will reflect your 'gut feelings' and your ability to discriminate between helpful and unhelpful emotions. Balance shows self-respect and respect for others. You will be outgoing, cheerful, relaxed and spontaneous, demonstrating emotional warmth.

An unbalanced Solar Plexus Chakra will show either very weak or very strong colours. These colours may be dark shades – black, brown or grey or a strong, dull red. When weakened, this chakra will reflect depression, insecurity, fear and poor digestion. Overactivity may make you judgmental, a workaholic, a perfectionist and resentful of authority.

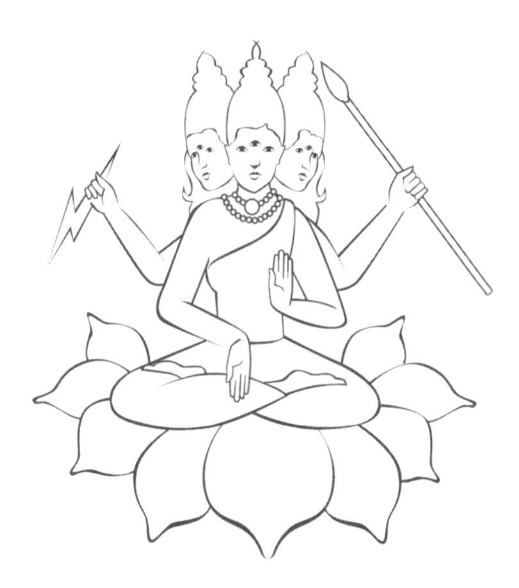

Scanning my Solar Plexus Chakra

Develop your intuition with this exercise. Make a tight fist with one hand – imagine it is your Solar Plexus, all knotted up! Imagine holding that tightness all day, every day. What does it mean to you? Is it fighting, holding on, aggressive acts, defence, anger or self-protection? Now unlock and relax your fist. Shake your hand vigorously. Let both your hands rest openly in your lap. How would your Solar Plexus feel if it was relaxed? Imagine what it would be like if everyone was like this, with open loving, caring hands and Solar Plexus Chakra.

Exercise 12 SENSING MY SOLAR PLEXUS ENERGY

CD REFERENCE TRACK 2 (OPTIONAL) (TO FOLLOW THE SCRIPT, TURN TO PAGE 110)

- **To begin,** lie down and relax. Keeping your eyes closed, push your fingers into your Solar Plexus area. What does it feel like? Relax, placing your hands by your sides.
- **Now begin to focus inwardly** upon this chakra's energy. Increase that focus. After a few minutes move one hand slowly around the area of your Solar Plexus Chakra, both within the auric field and on the body.
- **Notice whether your energy feels different** close into the body or further away. You may feel warmth/cold, lightness/heaviness, vibration/stillness, a colour, dense areas, vibrant areas or other sensations.
- **Remember what you feel,** so that you can record it on the following page.
- **Take a deep breath**, stretch, roll onto one side of your body and sit up slowly.
- **Now consider** the questions on page 102.

My sensing my solar plexus energy experience

Date ______________________ Signature ______________________

This exercise was: Easy / Hard / Took a while to get used to it

What did I sense? (tick or expand on what you felt)

Heat ______________________ Cold ______________________

Lightness ______________________ Heaviness ______________________

Vibration ______________________ Stillness ______________________

A colour ______________________

Dense areas ______________________

Does this mean my Solar Plexus Chakra energy is clogged/underactive? Yes / No

Do I need to activate it with colour-breathing golden yellow? Yes / No
(if your answer is Yes, please do so)

Vibrant areas ______________________

Does this mean my Solar Plexus Chakra energy is balanced? Yes / No

Did my Solar Plexus Chakra energy seem overactive? Yes / No

Do I need to calm it with colour-breathing violet? Yes / No
(if your answer Yes, go to Colour-Breathing a Rainbow on page 77, exchanging yellow for violet at the Solar Plexus level)

Other sensations? Describe ______________________

Checking my Solar Plexus is balanced

This exercise uses a pendulum to check whether your Solar Plexus Chakra is balanced. As recommended on page 18, try to build up empathy and confidence in your pendulum, so that it can be used reliably to determine degrees of activity in each of your chakras.

Remember to avoid holding the pendulum over a chakra, particularly if it is a crystal one – instead, point a finger of the other hand toward and near the chakra in question. This ensures that the pendulum doesn't falsify the reading.

Below are just some of the questions you may ask. Or how about asking if you need aromatherapy or sound healing exercises? Perhaps you need yoga or other balancing body movements? Can you think of more questions to enable you to go deeper? Any questions that you ask must have only 'Yes' or 'No' answers.

Exercise 13 DOWSING MY SOLAR PLEXUS CHAKRA

You will need: a pendulum, and a pen to record your results.

- **To begin,** remain focused and silent for a moment.
- **Then ask** the following questions:
  'Does this chakra require balancing?'
  'Is balance required on a physical level?'
  'Is balance required on a mental/emotional level?'
  'Is balance required on an energy level in my auric field?'

It is also relevant to ask:
'Is this chakra overactive or underactive?'
'Is colour-breathing required?'
'Is crystal balancing required?'
'Is a change in my lifestyle required?'

- **Record your pendulum results on** the opposite page (date and sign them), so that you can begin to see repeating (or varying) patterns of chakra activity. You may dowse just the Solar Plexus Chakra, or you have space there to record the condition of all your chakras, if you wish. You can also compare the effects that various methods shown in this book have upon the chakras, by dowsing before and after any balancing work. It becomes very exciting when you do this, because you can start to see positive results.
- **As an optional method of dowsing,** use a blank 'body outline' (see pages 238–49). Sign it (this is your 'witness' or energy imprint). With the understanding that this body outline represents you, rest your index finger on each chakra in turn. Hold the pendulum in the other hand, well away from your physical body. Ask the questions given above. Record and date your results.

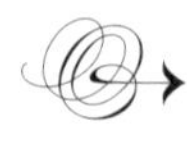

I'm not quite there yet Don't give up. Pendulum dowsing is a skill that can be very accurate as chakra 'diagnosis' and is a natural ability that many people once had in the past, but which we have now largely lost. Remember, practice makes perfect – but release your attachment to results. Maybe you would like to begin with a relaxation session? If so, Turn to Exercise 15: Complete Relaxation on page 110.

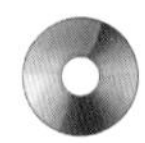

Work with the CD now Listen to CD reference Track 2 before you next attempt dowsing.

My dowsing my solar plexus chakra experience

Date ____________________ Signature ____________________

- Does this __________ Chakra require balancing? Yes / No
- Is balance required on a physical level? Yes / No
- Is balance required on a mental/emotional level? Yes / No
- Is balance required on an energy level in my auric field? Yes / No
- Is this __________ Chakra overactive? Yes / No
- Is colour-breathing required? Yes / No
- Is crystal balancing required? Yes / No
- Is a change in my lifestyle required? Yes / No
- Is this __________ Chakra underactive? Yes / No
- Is colour-breathing required? Yes / No
- Is crystal balancing required? Yes / No
- Is a change in my lifestyle required? Yes / No
- Ask any other questions that you wish to pose.

Circle the relevant states below:

Base Chakra	Balanced	Underactive	Overactive
Sacral Chakra	Balanced	Underactive	Overactive
Solar Plexus Chakra	Balanced	Underactive	Overactive
Heart Chakra	Balanced	Underactive	Overactive
Throat Chakra	Balanced	Underactive	Overactive
Third Eye Chakra	Balanced	Underactive	Overactive
Crown Chakra	Balanced	Underactive	Overactive

Recharging the Solar Plexus

The sun transduces (steps down) energies from outside our solar system and directs them to the planets. Esoterically the sun has been a metaphor for Divinity or Great Spirit – sunlight being 'Divine Light'. Native American traditions, as well as many other cultures, revere their cosmic connections, naming Father Sun, Mother Earth and Sister Moon. People who honour the sun in this way strengthen connections to their Solar Plexus Chakra – finding pleasure in the simple things of life, becoming less troubled by stress and having a tendency to be of a fiery nature, where negative emotions are released quickly. Ceremonies to give prayers and offerings to the sun are an everyday part of their culture. This exercise recharges your Solar Plexus with the power of the sun.

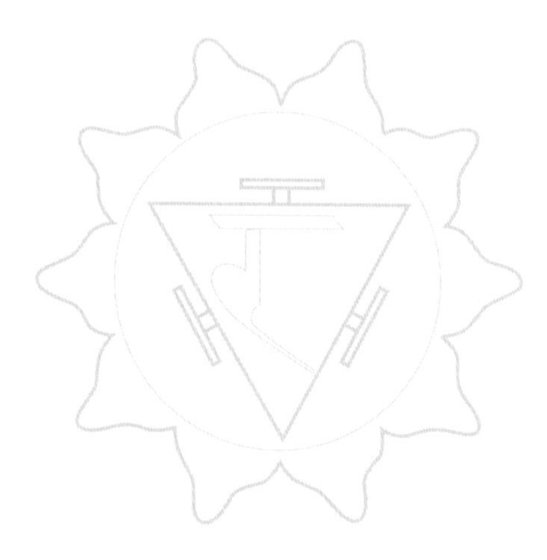

Exercise 14 BREATHING IN SOLAR ENERGIES

For this exercise you ideally need to meditate outside at dawn and watch the sun rise through half-closed eyes. Alternatively, stand before an open window. You may use any form of meditation that you are familiar with, or just go straight into the following visualization and colour-breathing.

- **Standing, breathe deeply** and place your hands on your solar plexus. Then, with each out-breath, extend your arms and hands toward the rising sun. Continue in this way for 13 breaths. Visualize each incoming breath as a beautiful golden yellow, the colour of the rising sun.
- **Then sit down** on a firm chair or in a cross-legged yoga posture and continue focusing upon your breath. Visualize each in-breath charged with a beautiful golden colour that revitalizes your Solar Plexus Chakra and then spreads to the whole of your body.
- **Once you feel your body glowing** with vitality, you will know that the visualization is working and complete.
- **Finish gently,** stretching your body and continuing with your day, recognizing with gracious appreciation that you are a little piece of the sun and that your solar meditation will sustain you.
- **Now consider** the questions on the following page. There is an extra page so that you can do the exercise more than once.

My breathing in solar energies experience

Date ______________________________

How well did I relax? Well / It was difficult / I couldn't relax at all

Was I outside at sunrise? Yes / No

Or did I stand before an open window? Yes / No

Was it easy to breathe in the energy of the sun? Yes / No

Did the colour-breathing help me focus on my Solar Plexus Chakra? Yes / No / A bit, but then I lost the focus / Don't know

How did this exercise affect me? ______________________________

____

____

____

____

____

____

Does my Solar Plexus Chakra feel more balanced? Yes / No / A bit/Don't know

My breathing in solar energies experience

Date ______________________________

How well did I relax? Well / It was difficult / I couldn't relax at all

Was I outside at sunrise? Yes / No

Or did I stand before an open window? Yes / No

Was it easy to breathe in the energy of the sun? Yes / No

Did the colour-breathing help me focus on my Solar Plexus Chakra? Yes / No / A bit, but then I lost the focus / Don't know

How did this exercise affect me? ______________________________

____

____

____

____

____

____

Does my Solar Plexus Chakra feel more balanced? Yes / No / A bit/Don't know

How to relax – fully!

I have taught this relaxation technique for more than 20 years to all my yoga and healer students. You will be lying very still, in order to relax and start 'communicating' with your chakras. Switch off your telephone and arrange not to be disturbed. This is your own quiet time; the CD track allocates 11 minutes, but once you are familiar with the process, you can extend it to 45 minutes or more. However, even relaxing for five minutes during a busy day is useful. You need to move into a state of deep relaxation, but not fall asleep. If you wish, you may place a 'grounding' stone (see page 62) beneath each foot. Wear loose clothing, if possible.

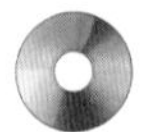

Exercise 15 COMPLETE RELAXATION

CD REFERENCE TRACK 2 (TO FOLLOW THE SCRIPT, SEE BELOW)

- **To begin,** lie on your blanket on your back and place a 'grounding' stone beneath each foot (optional). Close your eyes.
- **Be aware of the floor beneath your back.** Stretch your feet, then let them relax completely, slightly apart. Let your arms rest loosely at your sides, and move your head a little until your head and neck are in a comfortable position. Relax.
- **Take three really deep breaths** – breathe out slowly and relax totally. Your body will feel soft and warm. Your limbs will feel heavy, and it is not unusual to experience a floating sensation as you relax deeper.
- **Feel your arms and hands becoming limp** and heavy. Move your head gently from side to side to release any tension in your neck. Relax all the muscles of your face and scalp, and let the activity in your brain slow down.
- **Now focus inwardly on your Base Chakra** and legs. Let your legs and feet soften and sink down. Let your lower back relax a little more. Feel that through

your feet you are closely connected with the Earth, and allow the strength and energy of the Earth element to flow upward to clear any disharmony in your Base Chakra.

- **Focus inwardly on your Sacral Chakra.** Let your hips, buttocks, sexual organs and pelvis relax. Feel that through this chakra you can draw the cleansing power of Water to clear any disharmony.
- **Focus inwardly on your Solar Plexus Chakra.** Relax all your digestive organs, and soften the middle part of your back. Feel that through this chakra you can connect with the positive energies of the sun and draw in the power of Fire to clear any disharmony.
- **Focus inwardly on your Heart Chakra.** Relax and let the activity of your heart and lungs slow down. Experience waves of deep relaxation washing over you. Feel that through this chakra you can draw into your heart the freedom and empowerment of the Air element to clear any disharmony.
- **Allow the elemental quality of Spirit** to flow upward from your Heart Chakra to your throat and neck. Let a clear white light flow to the top of your head, dispelling any disharmony. Then gently let this light flow down and around your body, right to your feet. Wait a while in a lovely relaxed state.
- **To finish your relaxation,** begin to breathe a little deeper for some minutes. Deeper breathing integrates the elements of Earth, Water, Fire, Air and Spirit in your body. Return to everyday consciousness, sit up very slowly and take the rest of the day at an unhurried pace. Now record your experience in the space provided on page 112.

Later, when you feel ready to do so, you may also work on the Solar Plexus Chakra with any of the other balancing methods mentioned on other pages of this book. Consult the chart on page 83 to ascertain which aromatherapy oil to use, which yoga postures, colour breathing, and so on.

My complete relaxation experience

Date ______________________ Time ______________________

Before I started this relaxation I felt ______________________

____

____

____

____

During the relaxation I experienced ______________________

____

____

____

____

____

After the relaxation I felt ______________________

____

____

____

____

____

THE HEART CHAKRA: ANAHATA

Work with your chakras now Before you read further, turn to Exercise 16: Sensing and Drawing my Heart Chakra on page 130.

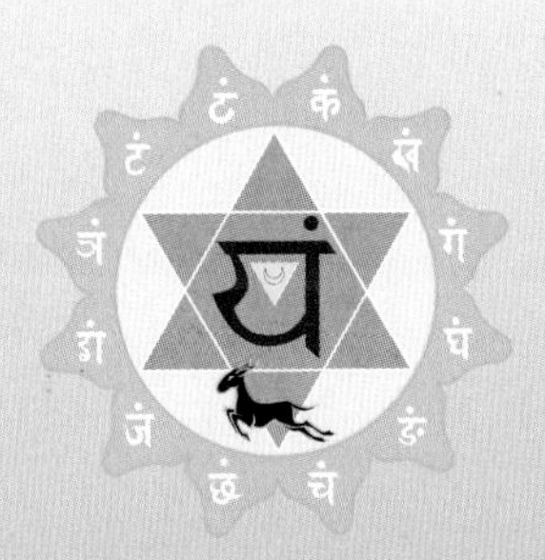

About my Heart Chakra

Keypoints: Resonates with the Air element and the colour crimson red, for the physical heart, and green for the chakra. In a healthy balance of this chakra we give empowerment, empathy and unconditional love to other people, as well as interacting in a caring way for the creatures and environment of our planet.

The fourth chakra, the Heart, is our inner power – harmony here allows us to break away from limiting external control. The Sanskrit name, *Anahata*, means 'the unstruck or unbeaten sound', which is the primordial source of all sound.

When you are on a path of personal growth, unconditional love and compassion develop through the Heart Chakra. You can encourage this within yourself by random acts of kindness. You will never regret making a commitment to work on this chakra. On one level, your dedication to the exercises in this book is designed to realign your state of wellness as preventative medicine. On another level, if you consistently align yourself to the Heart Chakra, you will make a swift discovery of a fundamental change that filters through your entire being. The presence you create will become noticeable to others in your life – a transcendence will occur.

The physical heart may be balanced with the colour of bright grass-green, and you can then bring in a soft pink for the chakra. If you are using crystals, first hold a cleansed aventurine to the Heart Chakra, then a rose quartz.

The Heart Chakra as lotus

Sometimes this chakra is visualized as a beautiful lotus flower: red for energy, pink for love, white for purity. When using a lotus (like a water-lily) as your visualization, consider this is a flower that began its life in the muddy 'waters of emotion' and rose magnificently to blossom above the water in the light. Imagine its petals opening up, as an inner radiance fills your being; remain in this space, immersing yourself in the experience. Then close each petal with love and care as you end your visualization.

CHART OF THE HEART CHAKRA

Colour of influence	Light and bright green
Complementary light colour	Magenta
Colour to calm	Pink
Physical location	Centre of chest on the sternum
Physiological system	Circulatory, lymphatic and immune systems
Endocrine system	Thymus
Key issues	Passion, tenderness, inner child and rejection issues
Inner teaching	Developing unconditional love and compassion
Energy action	Reception and distribution of unconditional love energy
Balancing crystals	Watermelon tourmaline, rose quartz, rhodocrosite, green aventurine
Balancing aromatherapy oils	Rose, melissa, neroli
Balancing herbal teas	Mix of lemon balm (melissa), hawthorn, rose petals and hips and raspberry leaf
Balancing yoga position (*asana*)	Bhujangasana (cobra), Janusirsasana (forward bend), Matsyasana (fish)
Mantra/tone	YAM in note of F (sounds like 'yarm')
Helpful musical instruments/music	Classical violin or piano sonatas, particularly by Mozart
Planet/astrological sign/natural House	Venus/Mercury/Libra/Virgo/seventh: partnerships/sixth: health
Reiki hand position	Two palms on the upper chest, then lift the hands off and place in a T-shape, with upper palm across the Heart Chakra and lower palm beneath it on the centre line
Power animal (Native American tradition)	All mammals

Body/Heart Chakra connections

The Heart Chakra influences our physical heart and lungs, respiratory system, circulatory and immune systems. At the back it is connected to the fourth thoracic vertebra, and at the front to the centre of the chest. It is common knowledge that our heart works like a pump, oxygenating blood. But the Heart Chakra also pumps energy in and out of our auric body, circulating it through the nadis.

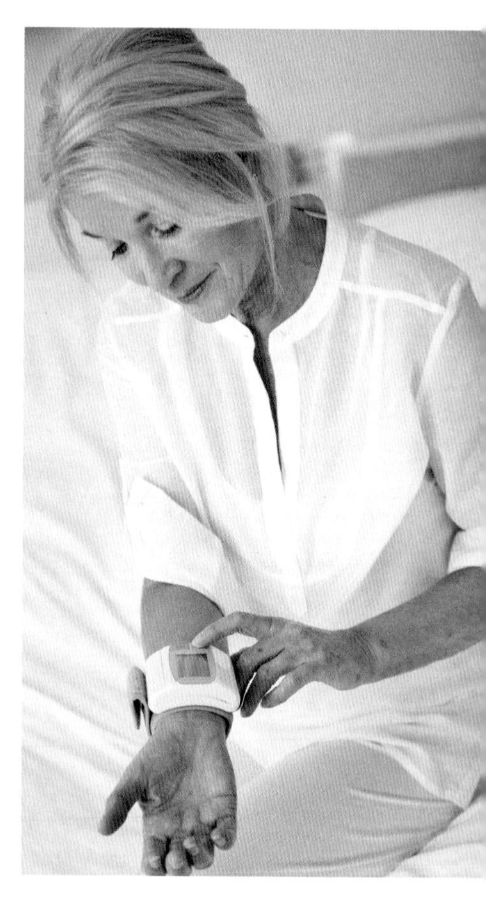

The body/mind connection

The constant action of the physical heart is marvellous, pumping more than 2.5 million litres (4.4 million pints) of blood a year, and coping with regular sport/exercise in normal circumstances. But it does respond adversely to stress and strain. Looking at the body/mind connection, a heart attack is a way for our body to demonstrate that we are overextending ourselves, paying too much attention to material, external and shallow aspects of our lives. Instead, can we express ourselves, and our love to others, and move on from hurtful situations to a state of equilibrium? Likewise, high blood pressure (which can be a precursor to a coronary) may be brought about by repressed anger and strong emotions, restricting the natural synchronization of the circulatory system – and cutting us off from letting our 'heart feelings' show. Maybe we feel we want to protect or hide our emotions because they are painful.

Continuing this body/mind connection, there is a logic in exploring the following clinical conditions, fibrositis, arthritis, pain or stiffness of the muscles or joints, because each may indicate rigidity in mental attitudes. There is a consequent stagnation of energy flow through the limbs, so you need to exercise more, balance the Heart Chakra and those chakras nearest the seat of the problem, to encourage self-love. Releasing emotional issues and improving breathing may also help bronchitis, which suggests repressed anger and the need to 'get things off your chest'. Remember that physiological signals are often an indication of something that has been held in your energy field for a long time.

“Believe in the impossible – visionary sight is our birthright.”

Work with your chakras now Turn to Exercise 18: Japanese Dō-In Energy Balancing on page 136, and start some simple movement techniques.

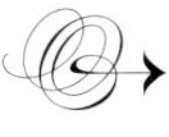

I'm not quite there yet Turn back to Exercise 3: Swallowing the Inner Smile on page 41. Remember, a smile is the cheapest facelift you can get!

The energy of my Heart Chakra

Within the auric field the Heart Chakra is linked to a secondary chakra, the Thymus or Higher Heart, in the centre of the chest. Medical science now accepts that the nearby minor thymus gland plays an important part in our immune system and in helping to regulate growth.

Some yogic teachings also associate the Heart Chakra with an additional spiritual heart centre just below, which develops as we remember our reason for incarnation. It is traditionally called the Kalpatree Chakra, Ananda-Kanda or, in modern terms, the Heart Seed. The associated colours of light to balance these chakras are pink-violet for the Thymus and yellow-gold for the Kalpatree.

It may surprise you to know that your hands are part of the flow of Heart Chakra energies too, for it is through them that we can experience the gift of touch. For example, when we sit or stand in a circle holding hands with a group of people, we move a constant wave of energy around the circle. It comes into one person's left hand, goes across the chest and is passed out via the right hand. This is just another instance of how we are all connected.

Life is an unfolding journey, and we rarely grow if we shut ourselves off from other people, who can reflect so much back to us. It is one of the ways we learn life's lessons. Again, the body/mind connection teaches us. Look at your feet, asking, 'What direction do I want to go in?' Look at your hands, asking, 'What are they really expressing?' Look at your face: what is your smile really saying?

When your heart energy is balanced, you may find yourself in energetic rapport with another person, based on complete understanding of one another. You are 'on the same wavelength' – literally, resonating together. People whom we describe as 'charismatic' have a well-balanced Heart Chakra and draw others toward them like a warming fire.

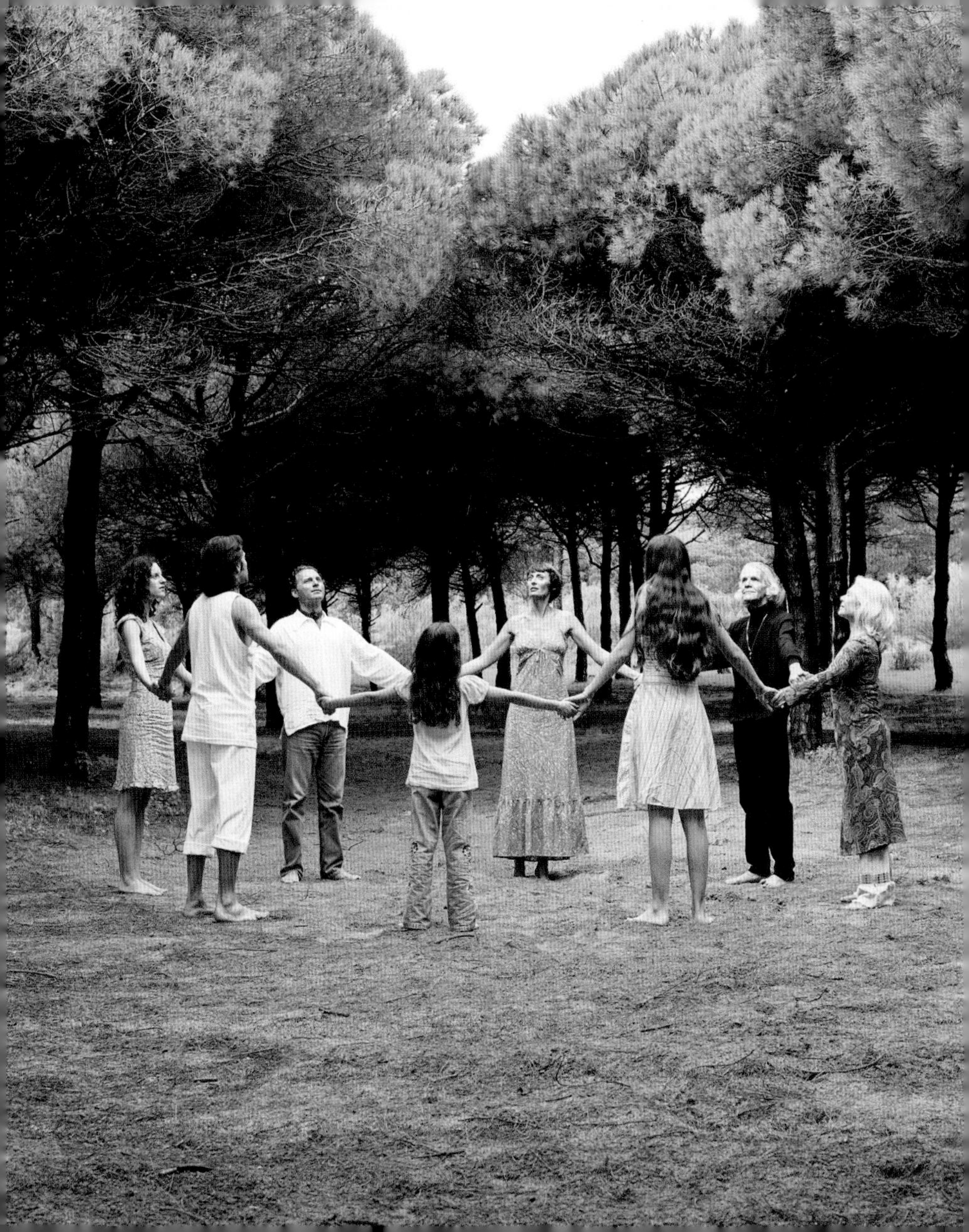

Yogic life lessons

The yogic symbol for the Heart Chakra is a circle surrounded by 12 green petals bearing Sanskrit letters for specific sounds. The 12 traditional lessons of life represented by this chakra are: lustfulness, fraudulence, indecision, repentance, hope, anxiety, longing, impartiality, arrogance, incompetence, discrimination and defiance. These lessons, concentrated at this chakra, have much to teach us about its function. They challenge us to overcome adversity, rising above our lower nature into the vibrations of the higher chakras.

According to these ancient esoteric yoga teachings, the Heart Chakra, in the centre of the Seven-Chakra System, is a 'gateway'. Locked below it are the energies of the first three chakras, which are primarily concerned with establishing our physical presence on Earth. Above it are the chakras more concerned with Spirit. When someone has worked sufficiently with all their challenging aspects, the Heart Chakra unlocks the gate to spiritual development. Energies then flow through an awakened spiritual heart to the higher chakras above it, where the core essence of humanity is destined to evolve and co-create a newly realized superconsciousness.

Love of Nature

In our hurry to fill the day with our 'doings' we have become quite separate from the world of Nature, seeing it as something out there to be enjoyed at weekends. Yet we too are part of the natural world, and every thought, every action we take, has an effect upon it. This occurs particularly through the Heart Chakra – where there is a need to take time to tend our 'inner garden'. When we work enthusiastically with this centre for positive personal growth, we discover that it leads us into 'seeing' that we are part of a greater picture. When we sustain this relationship, the wider cosmic field of life and Light becomes apparent.

What influences my Heart Chakra?

We have seen how, on a physical level, the circulation of air and oxygenated blood through the body are harmonized by the balanced functioning of this chakra, and that energy blockages may manifest as heart or lung disease. The flow of lymph is also closely linked to this area of the physical body. On a subtle-energy level, when the heart and its associated chakras (particularly the Thymus Chakra) are fully balanced, the physical body comes into a state where its basic needs are met. There is nothing more to do, for the heart is a marvellous organ that normally takes care of itself.

But on yet another level, heart care is people care! Now the real work of this chakra begins: the development of hope, forgiveness, peace, acceptance, openness, harmony and contentment.

“Smile into your heart.
This could prove to be the single most powerful act you can make to assist in self-healing.”

All these are aspects of unconditional divine love that we express toward ourselves and others.

The power of positive thinking

Wherever there is pain, ache or discomfort, place your hand upon the area. Medical research has proven that if positive thought is directed to any part of the body, blood flow increases and healing processes are initiated or improved through the enhanced circulation. In addition, circulate unconditional love by drawing it into your body with each breath, from whatever you feel is the source of divine love, within your own spiritual tradition. *Focus intently on your hands.* As they become much warmer, you will know that unconditional love is being transmitted into the area of discomfort. *Smile, and feel the release passing into your physical heart and out through the Heart Chakra.*

Holistic therapies show us that we are not fighting a battle with dis-ease.

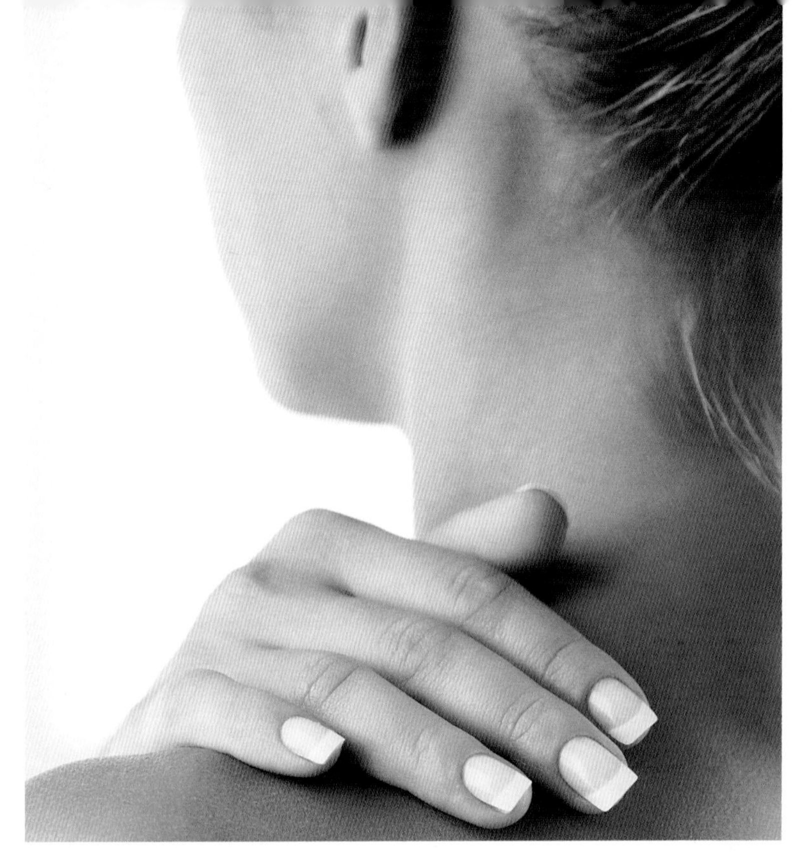

Nor should we become angry or despondent because of what we see as our limitations. When I give workshops, I teach that love is the only emotion that has ever made a positive difference to life. So never think of any part of your body as a nuisance because it is not completely healthy – *always* give praise for its marvellous intricacy, and direct loving thoughts toward it.

Adjust your perception, and be mindful of how you refer to certain body conditions: you don't want to fix dis-ease in your whole body/mind complex. For example, never say, 'I am an asthmatic' (instead, 'At present my physical body has asthma') or 'I am a diabetic' (instead, 'At present my physical body has diabetes'). Attitude of mind is a very important messenger for your body.

Balancing my Heart Chakra

Crystals and aromatherapy using rose essential oil are both excellent ways to balance the Heart Chakra. Rose has a sympathetic resonance with both the female and male reproductive systems, because it may contain plant hormone precursors.

Crystals

Here is a beneficial method that I have used many times with those who respond well to crystal energy. Begin by cleansing and dedicating your crystals, as suggested on page 62. Choose a green crystal to balance the physical heart – aventurine, green calcite or amazonite – and place it over your heart for a short while.

Then make a simple crystal layout of a six-pointed star. Ideally you will need six pink crystals, such as rose quartz or rhodocrosite, or six clear quartz tumbled stones, which will give you an overall boost and balance. Lie supine on your blanket and place a crystal on each side of your knees and one at your head – this forms the triangle of upward-flowing energies. Then place a crystal on each side of your shoulders and one

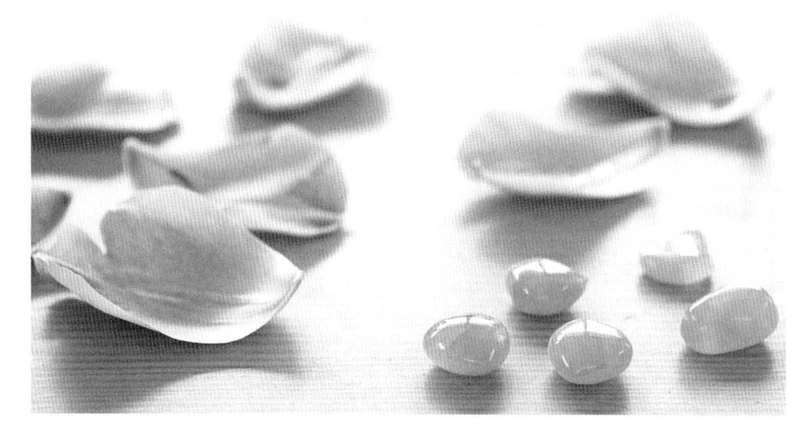

between your feet – this forms the triangle of downward-flowing energies.

Together the two triangles make the Heart Star of Harmonization and attract into your space – if you wish to call upon him/her – your guardian angel or the Archangel Chamuel and the angels of love who bring Christ Consciousness. Relax within the Heart Star of Harmonization crystal layout, and absorb the 'gifts' being brought to you through the crystals.

Aromatherapy using rose essential oil

It is believed that rose was the first-ever essential oil to be distilled by the Arab physician Avicenna in 11th-century Persia. He was probably attempting to produce alchemical gold by heating a combination of red and white rose petals in water – but made an essential oil instead! Rose oil is usually produced today as highly concentrated 'attar of rose'. Rose was traditionally known as an aphrodisiac; rose petals scattered on the nuptial bed have now been replaced by paper petals at weddings. Treatment from a qualified aromatherapist using rose and perhaps other essential oils aids postnatal depression and general anxiety. Rosewater is especially good for skincare.

A lovely way to connect with the natural energies of rose is to place a fragrant real rose (of whatever colour you wish) before you, then meditate upon its beauty. However, the use of rose oil is intended to stimulate the subtle-energy fields that link to the heart, thus bringing balance so that you can find the mystical 'alchemical gold' at the heart-centre. You can do this with aromatherapy, or by showing everyday concern for those nearest and dearest to you, as well as random acts of kindness to strangers. As the heart centre becomes more loving and 'open', you naturally shift your life emphasis away from the lower self to altruistic concerns and development of your spiritual self.

For details of how to use this and other essential oils, see page 94.

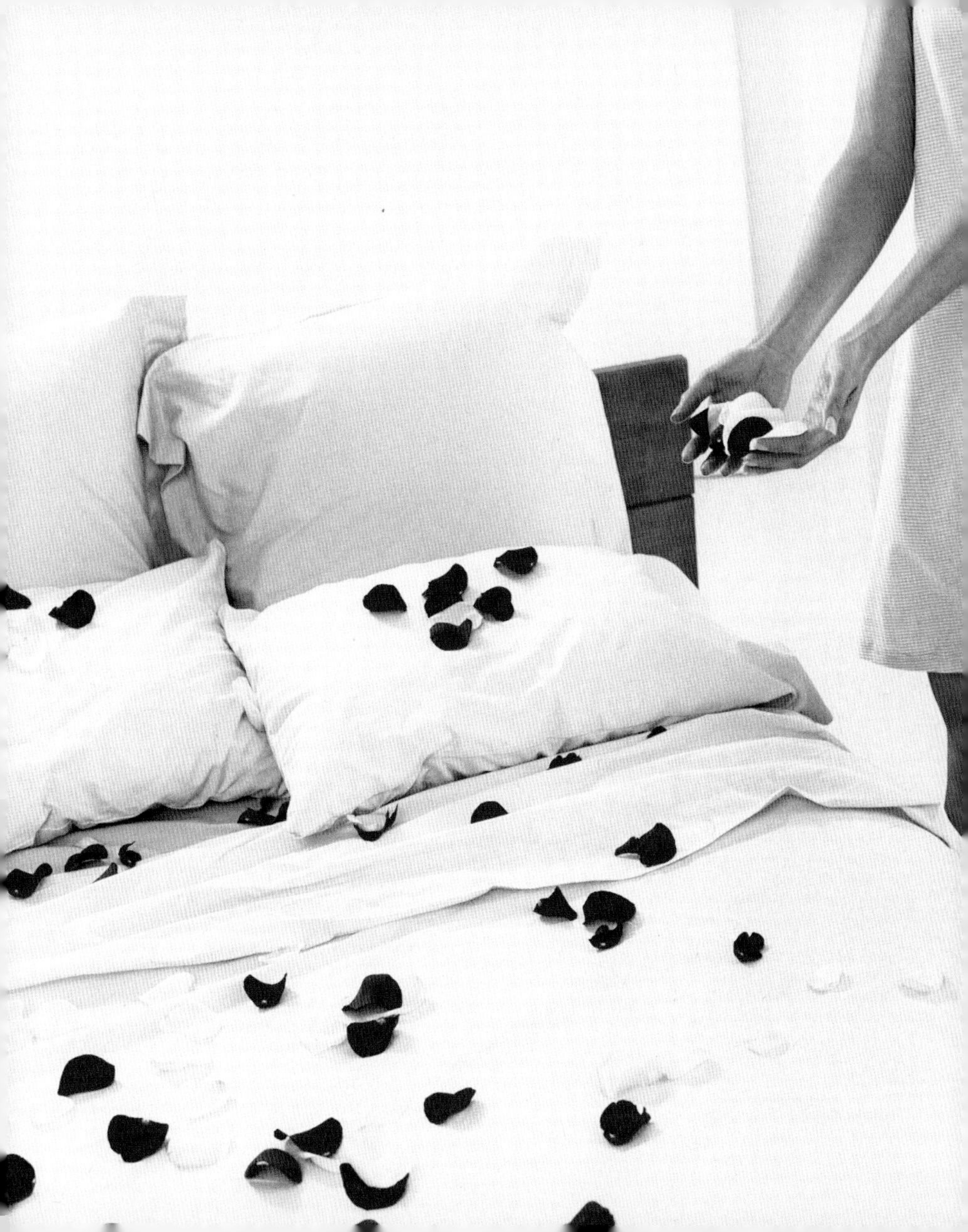

Understanding stress

Despite our best efforts to look after ourselves, the midpoint balance of the Heart Chakra in the Seven-Chakra System is sometimes challenged. Stress is a major contributory factor to any imbalanced chakras that affect our body functions and our state of wellness. So check yourself out from the head down.! Do any of the following manifest themselves in your physical body?

- Headaches, dizziness
- Insomnia
- Panic attacks
- Blurred vision
- Difficulty in swallowing
- Aching neck muscles, stiff jaw
- A susceptibility to infection
- High blood pressure, cardiovascular disorders
- Overbreathing, asthma, palpitations
- Excessive sugar in the blood
- Nervous indigestion, stomach ulcers
- Backache, aching muscles generally
- Nervous rashes and allergies
- Excessive sweating
- Mucous colitis, irritable bowel syndrome, constipation, diarrhoea
- Sexual difficulties, hormonal imbalances, inability to conceive.

Realize that, from a metaphysical point of view, all body dysfunction has first permeated the auric field, entered the chakra and nadi systems and finally come to rest in (usually the weakest part of) the physical body.

A healer will not endeavour to shift physical symptoms, but these will often lessen as the whole body/mind/spirit complex comes into balance.

Work with your chakras now Turn to Exercise 20: Dowsing my Heart Chakra on page 141, to check that this chakra is balanced.

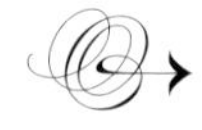

I'm not quite there yet Listen to CD reference Track 2 again, for relaxation is the key to harmony.

What can I do about stress?

You need to recognize that too many lifestyle changes at the same time put a major strain upon the body. By 'lifestyle changes' we mean milestones in life, such as divorce, the death of a loved one, personal injury or illness, a change of job, moving house, getting married, having a baby, an abusive relationship or encounters with law-enforcement or other authorities. Try the following steps to reduce your stress levels:

- Take action before you 'crack up' or become ill. Recognize your tiredness and exactly how much of it you can tolerate.
- Change your environment: get away from the situation that causes you stress, if you can. It may save your life.!
- Detox regularly. Avoid alcoholic drink and drugs.
- 'Switch off' for a while during your working day.

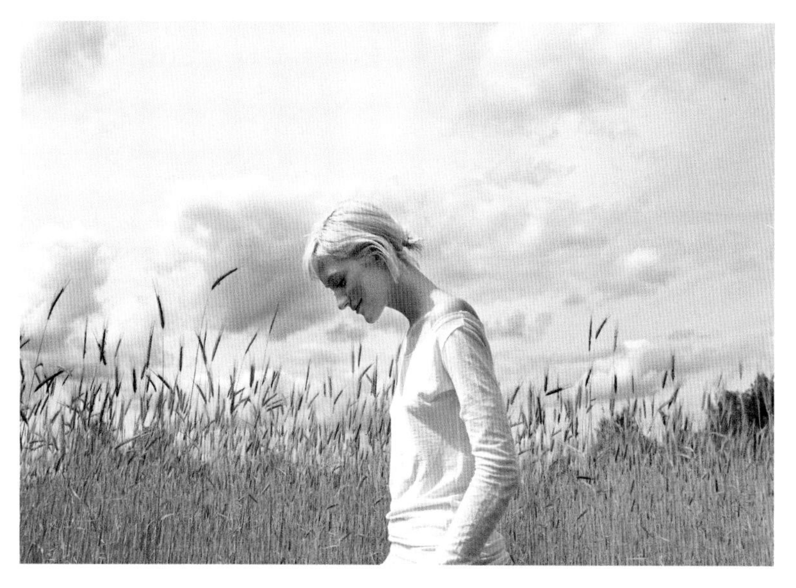

- Keep fit and eat healthily.
- Learn a relaxation technique and how to breathe fully (see Exercise 15: Complete Relaxation on page 110).
- Be aware of your energy field, all your chakras and how to keep them in balance. Use Japanese Dō-In (see Exercise 18 on page 136).
- Treat yourself to a relaxing health treatment, sauna or weekend break.
- Walk outside more often and enjoy Nature.
- Take up hobbies and leisure activities, such as yoga, t'ai chi ch'uan or other energy techniques.
- Gracefully accept whatever good and positive things are around you.
- Examine your feelings of stress, and don't let them alarm you. When you have recovered, use the experience to deepen your understanding of other people.
- Help others, and be an example of how to 'cope with stress *without* distress'.

Work with your chakras now Turn to Exercise 18: Japanese Dō-In Energy Balancing on page 136.

Work with your chakras now Turn to Exercise 17: Heart Chakra Visualization on page 133, or listen to CD reference Track 3 to meditate.

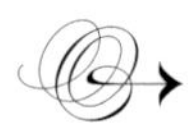

I'm not quite there yet Turn to Exercise 19: Colour-Breathing the Thymus Chakra on page 139

HEART CHAKRA EXERCISES

The following exercises develop the Heart Chakra or Anahata. It is the centre of your innermost love, which ideally is expressed to others unconditionally. You will use a self-assessment about the power of love, plus 'colour-breathing' and developing intuition and meditation skills with the CD, among other ways of rebalancing this important chakra.

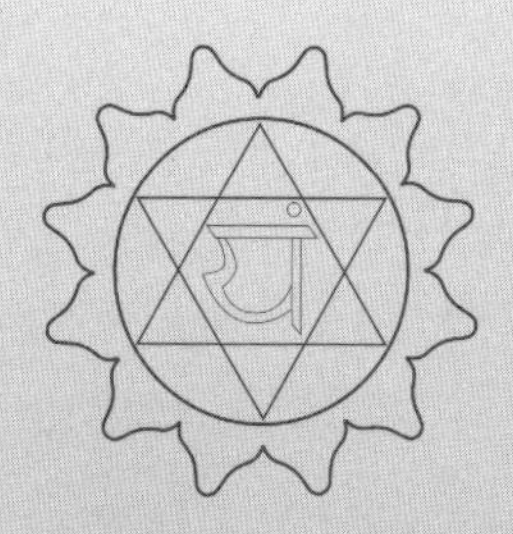

Developing intuition

Do this exercise before reading beyond this page. It will become a record of your Heart Chakra – showing how content or insecure you are – to which you can refer back in order to chart your progress.

Exercise 16 SENSING AND DRAWING MY HEART CHAKRA

You will need: a set of coloured pencils or pens (all colours, including magenta); keep the book open, ready to colour in the body outline opposite, which represents you (sign and date it before you begin).

- **To begin,** take five minutes sitting in a quiet place, breathing slowly, relaxing and closing your eyes. Now start to sense your body and your aura. Release any emotions that arise. Forget anything you have ever heard or read about chakras and auras. You are simply sensing how your own unique energies are flowing at present. Check from your feet up to your head to pick up any little clues that your body is giving you. Sense your auric energy field around you as well. Now focus upon your Heart Chakra area. What is it telling you? What can you sense? Does it feel free, flowing, harmonious? Or is an old pain or trauma held there? Does this area feel fluid and open – or have you shut off all feelings and thoughts of this chakra?
- **When you feel ready,** open your eyes and – immediately and without thinking – quickly colour in the Heart Chakra area and any other parts of the body (and the surrounding page) as you wish. There is no right or wrong place to apply the colour: it is entirely up to you.
- **Read the interpretation** on page 132 after completing this exercise.

I'm not quite there yet Listen to CD reference Track 2, if you don't feel relaxed enough to do this exercise yet; come back to it later on.

My sensing and drawing my heart chakra experience

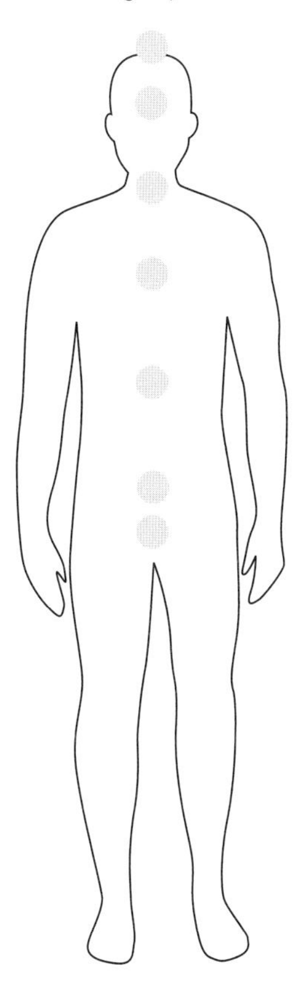

Date ______________________ Signature ______________________

Assessing my results for Exercise 16

A balanced Heart Chakra will show strong and vibrant colours of red, green or pink. It will reflect your inner feelings of self-worth, contentment and the ability to give empathy, unconditional love and compassion.

An unbalanced Heart Chakra will show either very weak or very strong colours. These may be dark shades – black, brown or grey or a strong, dull red. When weakened, it will reflect depression, insecurity or 'a broken heart'. Excessive activity may make you overreactive, intolerant and bombastic, or continually seeking loving relationships to balance yourself.

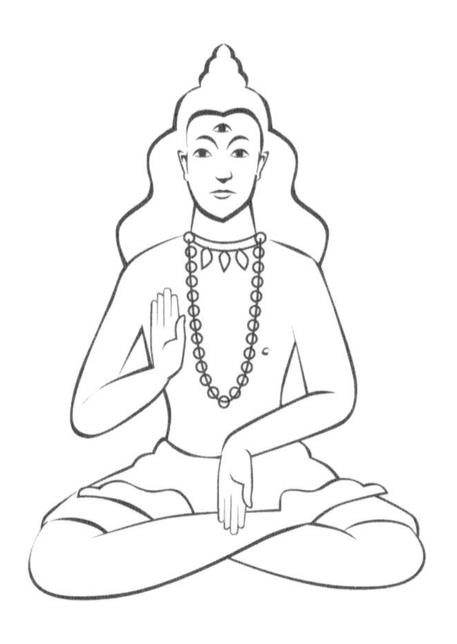

Meditative visualization

This is a meditative visualization to link you to Earth and Sky through the element of Air. If you have an oil vaporizer, use rose or rose geranium oil in it; alternatively, place a pink flower in a vase or hold a rose quartz crystal in your hand, putting you in touch with Heart Chakra energy frequencies.

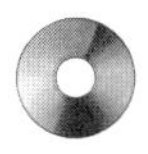

Exercise 17 HEART CHAKRA VISUALIZATION

CD REFERENCE TRACK 2 (OPTIONAL) (TO FOLLOW THE SCRIPT, TURN TO PAGE 110) **CD REFERENCE** TRACK 3 (TO FOLLOW THE SCRIPT, SEE BELOW)

You will need: a set of coloured pencils or pens.

- **To begin,** light a candle. Sit and relax, then close your eyes. Remember to keep your spine straight.
- **Breathe slowly and deeply,** feeling the expansion of your lungs. Listen to your beating heart.
- **Notice the expansion of your chest** as you breathe. Breathe in all aspects of the Nature element of Air, ranging from a strong gust of air to a soft breeze. Feel this air rush into your body and energize it with *prana*.
- **Connect to your Heart Chakra,** visualizing it as a beautiful pink lotus flower. Observe the flower closely. Notice whether it is a tightly shut bud or fully open. If it is open, what do you see inside?
- **Now visualize the place** where the lotus is growing. It needs water to grow and flower. So see the water, sky and whatever else is around. Are there more lotus flowers?
- **Focus on your own lotus,** the one you first visualized, as a single bloom. Notice whether it has changed, and whether you can now see its centre of golden stamens.

- **To finish,** ask the lotus to close its petals. Then put a circle of clear bright emerald-green light around it. As you do so, ask for the protection of your Heart Chakra with another circle of clear bright emerald-green light.
- **Finally,** put your right hand crosswise across your chest, followed by the left in the same manner.
- **Open your eyes** and blow out the candle.
- **As with all meditative visualizations,** it is a good idea to record your experiences on the next page, and to draw your lotus, if you wish.
- **Now consider** the questions on page 135.

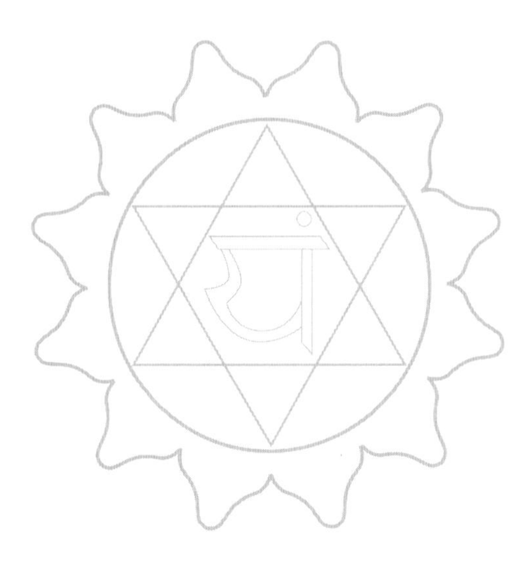

My heart chakra visualization experience

Date ______________________________

Was this exercise difficult ?: Yes / No / A little

How well did I visualize the lotus flower? ______________________________

____

____

What did it look like? ______________________________

____

____

What (if anything) could I see inside the lotus? ______________________________

____

____

What did I feel about this exercise? ______________________________

____

____

What did I learn from it? ______________________________

____

____

Daily exercise for total balance

This once-daily exercise is based on teachings stemming from the Tao of Shin Sen, an ancient collection of Dō-In exercises and the practice of them as a spiritual path. It was originally used by Zen monks over a wide area of China, Japan, Korea and Vietnam.

Exercise 18 JAPANESE DŌ-IN ENERGY BALANCING

- **To begin,** kneel on a mat with your hands resting lightly on your lap. Aim to keep your consciousness in the unlimited ocean of tranquillity of Oneness. Clap your hands together twice to purify your space. Rub your face all over with the palms of your hands. Then tap your face all over with your fingertips.
- **With lightly gripped fists,** tap your entire head lightly, as if they are bouncing off it. Use the side of the fist at the little finger. This stimulates all its physical and mental activities and the coordination of various physical and energy systems.
- **Pound the opposite shoulder** with one fist about 30 times. Repeat on the other side and at the back of your neck.
- **Kneel up and vigorously pound** with both fists as much of your back, buttocks and the backs of your legs as you can reach. Gently pound the centre of your chest to stimulate the thymus region.
- **Kneel down again.** Open your arms in front of you and vigorously tap with the fingertips of one hand up the inside of the other arm from fingers to shoulder, then round and down the outside of the arm, right to the fingertips. Repeat seven times on each arm.
- **With one palm over the other,** slowly and deeply massage the whole of the soft abdominal area in a clockwise action about 20 times.

- **Sit, stretching out your legs.** Vigorously tap with your fingertips from the toes up the inside of the leg to your groin, then round and down the side and back of the leg to the toes. Repeat seven times on each leg.
- **With the soles of your feet together,** hold them with your hands and breathe deeply seven times, harmonizing the energy flow.
- **Now consider** the questions on page 138.

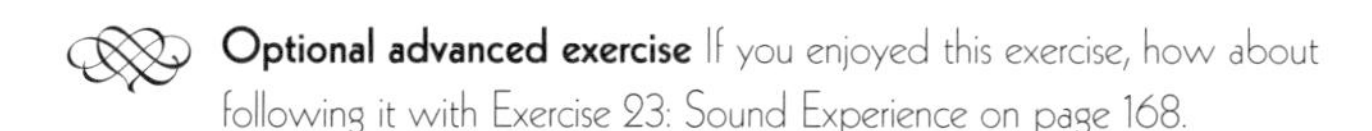

Optional advanced exercise If you enjoyed this exercise, how about following it with Exercise 23: Sound Experience on page 168.

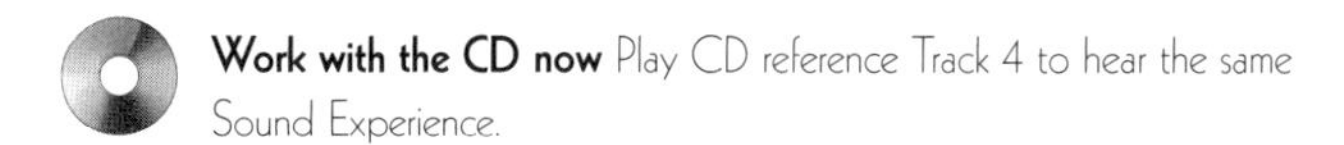

Work with the CD now Play CD reference Track 4 to hear the same Sound Experience.

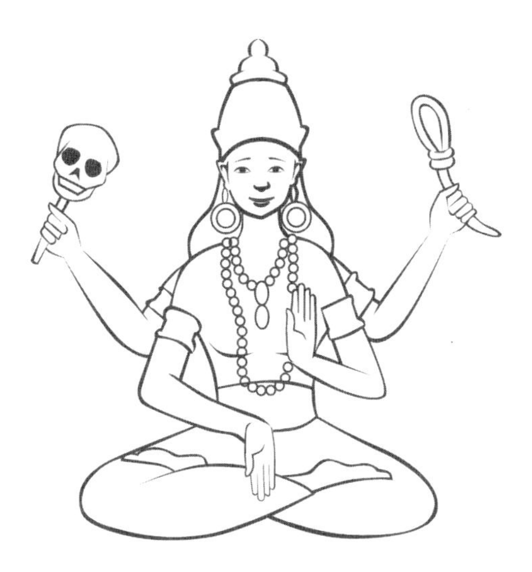

My Japanese dō-in energy balancing experience

Date ______________________ Time of day ______________________

What was my physical energy level before the exercise? ______________________

____

What was my physical energy level after the exercise? ______________________

____

What was my mental/emotional energy level before the exercise? ______________________

____

What was my mental/emotional energy level after the exercise? ______________________

____

What else did I feel? ______________________

____

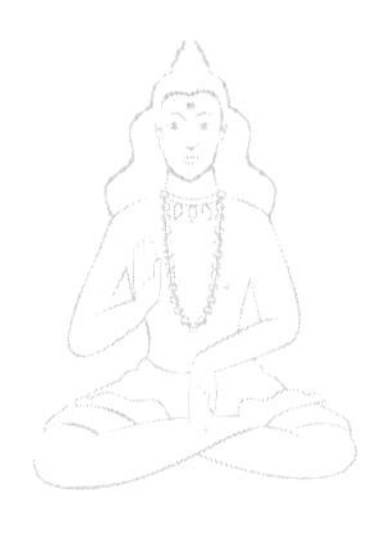

Recharging the Thymus Chakra

This exercise continues your colour-breathing visualization practice, improving the depth and quality of your breathing and bringing a particular emphasis upon the Heart Chakra region.

You need to be in a place where you will not be disturbed for between ten minutes and half an hour – indoors is okay, but it would be even better to be sitting outside in Nature.

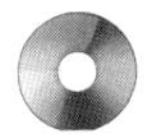

Exercise 19 COLOUR-BREATHING MY THYMUS CHAKRA

CD REFERENCE TRACK 2 (OPTIONAL) (TO FOLLOW THE SCRIPT, TURN TO PAGE 110)

- **To begin,** sit in an upright chair or a cross-legged yoga posture. Ensure that you are fully relaxed. Your spine must be as straight as possible and your chin pulled in, to straighten the back of your neck.
- **Close your eyes** and breathe slowly, visualizing your incoming breath as a clear, bright grass-green light. Breathe deeply for a few minutes, focusing on the Heart Chakra. Feel this coloured breath suffusing the area of your physical and subtle heart with beneficial new energy, helping to clear and balance it.
- **Now change the colour** of your breath to a pink/violet light, focusing on your Heart Chakra and the Thymus Chakra, just above it, for a few minutes. Feel this coloured breath suffusing the area of your physical and subtle heart with more energy, bringing wellness and inner peace.
- **Return to normal breathing** and, after some minutes, open your eyes.
- **Now consider** the questions on page 140.

My colour-breathing my thymus chakra experience

Date ______________________________

How well did I relax? Well / It was difficult / I couldn't relax at all

Did the colour breathing help me focus on my Heart Chakra?
Yes / No / A bit, but then I lost focus / Don't know

Did the colour-breathing help me focus on my Thymus Chakra?
Yes / No / A bit, but then I lost focus / Don't know

How did this exercise affect me? ______________________________

____

____

____

____

____

____

Does my Heart Chakra feel more balanced? Yes / No / A bit / Don't know

Checking my Heart Chakra is balanced

This exercise uses a pendulum to check whether your Heart Chakra is balanced. As recommended on page 18, try to build up empathy and confidence in your pendulum, so that it can be used reliably to determine degrees of activity in each of your chakras.

Remember to avoid holding the pendulum over a chakra, particularly if it is a crystal one – instead, point a finger of the other hand toward and near the chakra in question. This ensures that the pendulum doesn't falsify the reading.

Below are just some of the questions you may ask. Or how about asking if you need aromatherapy or sound healing exercises? Perhaps you need yoga or other balancing body movements? Any questions that you ask must have only 'Yes' or 'No' answers.

Exercise 20 DOWSING MY HEART CHAKRA

You will need: a pendulum, and a pen to record your results.

- **To begin,** remain focused and silent for a moment.
- **Then ask** the following questions:
  'Does this chakra require balancing?'
  'Is balance required on a physical level?'
  'Is balance required on a mental/emotional level?'
  'Is balance required on an energy level in my auric field?'

  It is also relevant to ask:
  'Is this chakra overactive or underactive?'

'Is colour-breathing required?'
'Is crystal balancing required?'
'Is a change in my lifestyle required?'

- **Record your pendulum results** on the opposite page (date and sign them), so that you can begin to see repeating (or varying) patterns of chakra activity. You may dowse just the Heart Chakra, or you have space there to record the condition of all your chakras, if you wish. You can also compare the effects that various methods shown in this book have upon the chakras, by dowsing before and after any balancing work. It becomes very exciting when you do this, because you can start to see positive results. There is an extra page overleaf so that you can do the exercise more than once.
- **As an optional method of dowsing,** use a blank 'body outline' (see pages 238–49). Sign it (this is your 'witness' or energy imprint). With the understanding that this body outline represents you, rest your index finger on each chakra in turn. Hold the pendulum in the other hand, well away from your physical body. Ask the questions given above. Record and date your results.

Later, when you feel ready to do so, you may also work on the Heart Chakra with any of the other balancing methods mentioned on other pages of this book. Consult the chart on page 115 to ascertain which aromatherapy oil to use, which yoga postures, colour breathing, and so on.

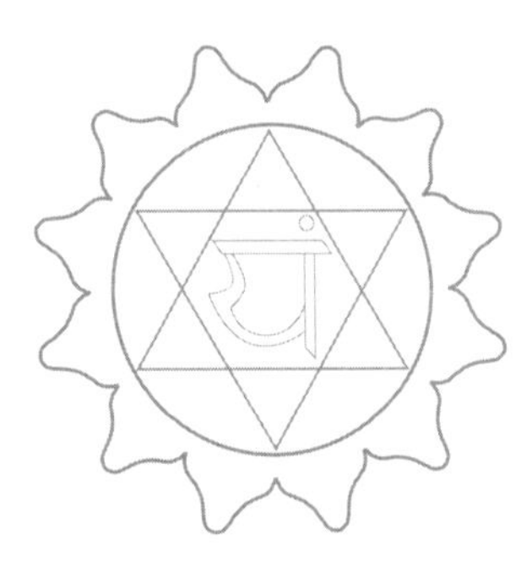

My dowsing my heart chakra experience

Date ______________________ Signature ______________________

- Does this __________ Chakra require balancing? Yes / No
- Is balance required on a physical level? Yes / No
- Is balance required on a mental/emotional level? Yes / No
- Is balance required on an energy level in my auric field? Yes / No
- Is this __________ Chakra overactive? Yes / No
- Is colour-breathing required? Yes / No
- Is crystal balancing required? Yes / No
- Is a change in my lifestyle required? Yes / No
- Is this __________ Chakra underactive? Yes / No
- Is colour-breathing required? Yes / No
- Is crystal balancing required? Yes / No
- Is a change in my lifestyle required? Yes / No
- Ask any other questions that you wish to pose.

Circle the relevant states below:

Base Chakra	Balanced	Underactive	Overactive
Sacral Chakra	Balanced	Underactive	Overactive
Solar Plexus Chakra	Balanced	Underactive	Overactive
Heart Chakra	Balanced	Underactive	Overactive
Throat Chakra	Balanced	Underactive	Overactive
Third Eye Chakra	Balanced	Underactive	Overactive
Crown Chakra	Balanced	Underactive	Overactive

My dowsing my heart chakra experience

Date ______________________ Signature ______________________

- Does this ____________ Chakra require balancing? Yes / No
- Is balance required on a physical level? Yes / No
- Is balance required on a mental/emotional level? Yes / No
- Is balance required on an energy level in my auric field? Yes / No
- Is this ____________ Chakra overactive? Yes / No
- Is colour-breathing required? Yes / No
- Is crystal balancing required? Yes / No
- Is a change in my lifestyle required? Yes / No
- Is this ____________ Chakra underactive? Yes / No
- Is colour-breathing required? Yes / No
- Is crystal balancing required? Yes / No
- Is a change in my lifestyle required? Yes / No
- Ask any other questions that you wish to pose.

Circle the relevant states below:

Base Chakra	Balanced	Underactive	Overactive
Sacral Chakra	Balanced	Underactive	Overactive
Solar Plexus Chakra	Balanced	Underactive	Overactive
Heart Chakra	Balanced	Underactive	Overactive
Throat Chakra	Balanced	Underactive	Overactive
Third Eye Chakra	Balanced	Underactive	Overactive
Crown Chakra	Balanced	Underactive	Overactive

THE THROAT CHAKRA: VISHUDDHA

 **Work with your chakras now** Before you read further, turn to Exercise 21: Sensing and Drawing my Throat Chakra on page 162.

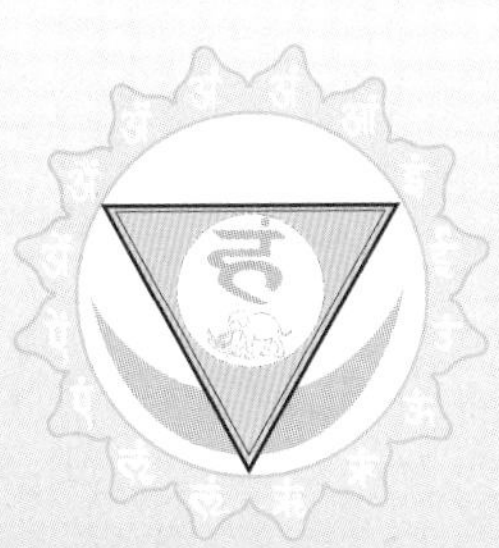

About my Throat Chakra

Keypoints: Resonates with the Ether element (akasha in Sanskrit) and the colour turquoise-blue; concerned with developing our self-expression, communication and will.

The fifth chakra, the Throat, is the centre of our personal expression and flexibility, enabling us to break away from limiting external control. The Sanskrit name, Vishuddha, means 'to purify'. At the fifth chakra we have the opportunity to purify the energies of all the lower chakras, so that they may pass through the narrow channel of the neck into the head.

This chakra develops speech, communication, song, telepathy and channelled information. Sound is the sense held within it, brought about by the Earth element at the Base Chakra dissolving in Water at the Sacral Chakra, leaving a sense of smell. The Water is then vaporized by Fire at the Solar Plexus, leaving a sense of taste. As Fire enters the Heart Chakra, the Air moves, leaving a sense of touch. When the Air enters the Throat, it becomes sound.

The crystal of choice to activate the Throat Chakra is blue topaz for spiritual insights and yellow topaz for physical energy. You do not need expensive gem-quality topaz; natural, uncut topaz, which is just as beneficial, can be obtained. Excellent balancing crystals are chrysocolla and turquoise; always try to get natural turquoise, not a reconstituted or a dyed stone. One way to use crystals is to place a small one in the notch of the collarbone, or two on either side of the neck, for 10–20 minutes for best effect.

To calm the Throat Chakra, consider sipping turquoise solarized water (see page 187 for its preparation). Using the resonant frequencies of light, the water becomes intentionally aligned with a minute homeopathic quantity of the turquoise frequency required by this chakra.

Work with your chakras now Turn to Exercise 22: Throat Chakra Visualization on page 165, to enjoy a relaxing meditation visualization.

CHART OF THE THROAT CHAKRA

Colour of influence	Turquoise-blue
Complementary light colour	Red
Colour to calm	Turquoise-blue, pale blue or pale green
Physical location	Between collarbone and larynx on the neck
Physiological system	Respiratory
Endocrine system	Thyroid and parathyroid
Key issues	Self-expression, communication and will
Inner teaching	To develop compassion and caring self-expression
Energy action	A bridge between the physical and spiritual
Balancing crystals	Turquoise, gem silica, chrysocolla
Balancing aromatherapy oils	Lavender, Roman chamomile (and rosemary, thyme, sage, unless pregnant)
Balancing herbal teas	Mix of echinacea, lobelia, elderberry, marshmallow, red sage, cleavers and honey
Balancing yoga position (*asana*)	Dhanurasana (bow), Simhasana (lion), Paschimottanasana (sitting forward bend)
Mantra/tone	HAM in the note of G (sounds like 'harm')
Helpful musical instruments/music	Flute
Planet/astrological sign/natural House	Jupiter/Mars/Sagittarius/Scorpio/ninth: intellect, eighth: death
Reiki hand position	Two palms gently over the throat
Power animal (Native American tradition)	All humanity

Body/Throat Chakra connections

The Throat Chakra is located on the front of the neck and at the corresponding part of the spine – the third cervical vertebra – at the back. This is where the body is narrowing and concentrating all its energies, to enable information to pass up through the neck to the brain. It is a major body 'highway' that can become overburdened and blocked; repeated physical infections of the throat may be an indicator of this.

This chakra is primarily linked to the thyroid, a large endocrine gland lying at the base of the neck, affecting cellular metabolism and growth stimulation. It also encourages the onset of puberty and sexual maturity, as well as acting as protection against infection. In addition it is linked to two parathyroid glands in the physical body, through the two secondary parathyroid chakras and two clavicle chakras. The hormones secreted by the parathyroids aid normal growth and the vital metabolism of calcium for our bone structure.

The whole of the ear/nose/throat connection, dealing with hearing and speech, and to some extent the respiratory system are also connected to this chakra. So for imbalances in these areas, which show up as dis-ease or discomfort, the Throat Chakra needs to receive healing. Additionally this is the region of your physical body where pollution – such as smoke, inappropriate food or drink – is ingested, and where words/sound/song are emitted.

Neck rotations Japanese-style

The following simple exercise releases tension that builds up in the 'bottleneck' of the body. Sit down, relax your shoulders and then rotate your head *slowly*. If you feel any tightness or pain, stop and massage the area with your fingertips. Then resume the rotations. If you feel dizzy, slow down the speed of rotation. Ensure that you rotate in each direction an equal number of times. Also consider practising Dō-In exercises, to keep your body and chakras balanced.

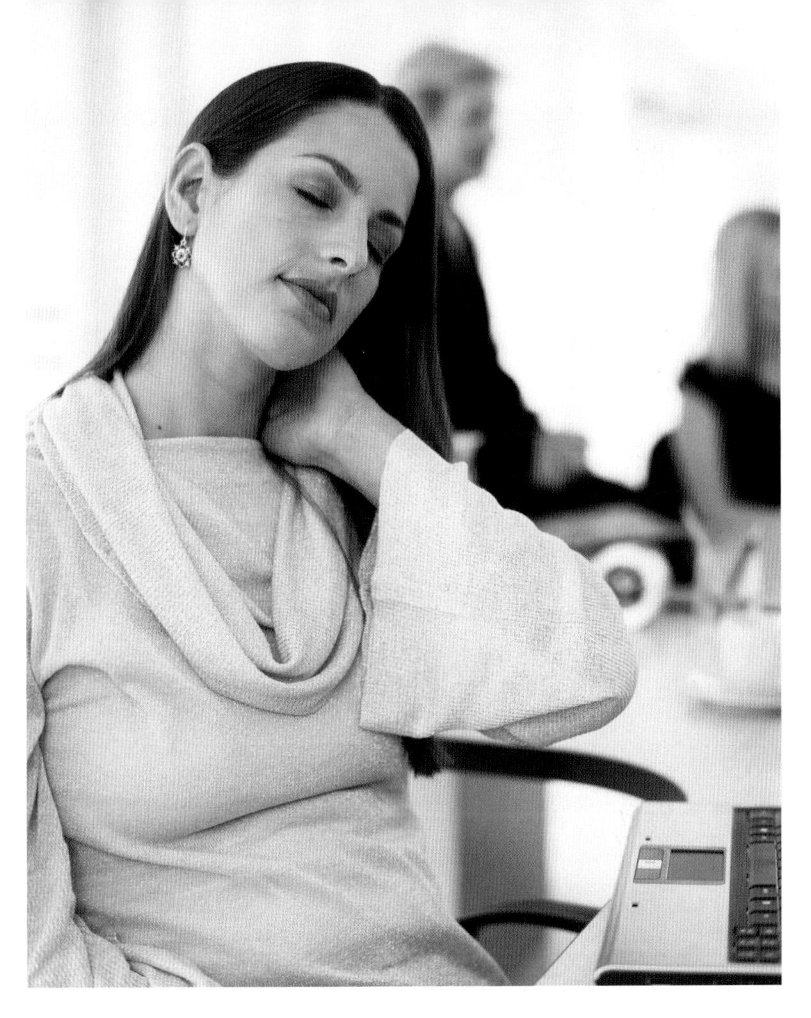

Work with your chakras now Turn to Exercise 18: Japanese Dō-In Energy Balancing on page 136, and remember to spend a little while on these exercises each day, and especially on the neck rotations given above, if you sit in front of a computer for long periods of time.

The energy of my Throat Chakra

The Throat is one of the most important chakras, for not only does it act as a vital 'bridge' on the highway between the physical body and the neck, as I have explained, but also as a bridge between different realities.

Generally the chakras are believed to become most energized or developed sequentially from Base to Crown. In this model of the development of the inner aspects of chakra energies, once the Throat Chakra is receptive, this highway takes us to a different land, another side of the 'River of Life', where access through the dimensions to spiritual realms is achievable.

Mysteriously supporting these other dimensions of soul and spirit is the nebulous Nature element of Ether. In the associated yoga symbol there are petals that are sometimes a smoky-blue, representative of Ether, together with an unyoked elephant, indicating the inherent strength and power that can be developed from this chakra.

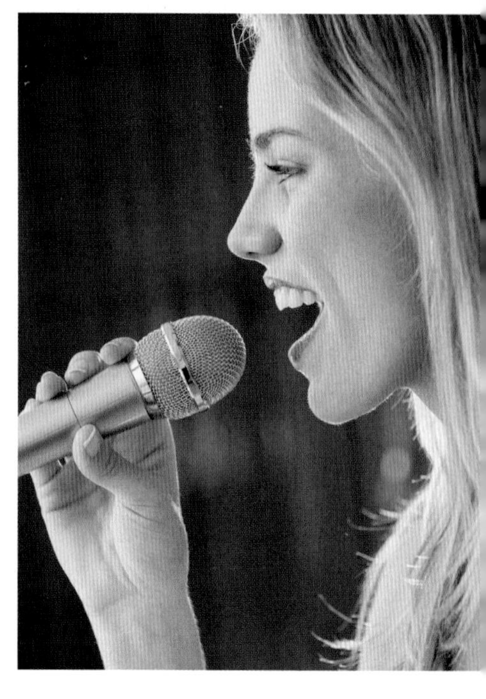

Connections between the Throat and Heart Chakras

The most obvious examples of positive Throat Chakra balance are singing, public speaking and acting. Singers usually have a well-developed Throat Chakra. When this chakra comes into balance, we are able to express ourselves and our love for others through our words.

The Throat Chakra is closely linked with the Heart Chakra, because there is a natural tendency arising in the Heart Chakra for loving words and song. Our intentions are imprinted upon the emanations from our voice, and analysis can confirm that we either have a good range of tones and harmonies or our voice is dull and boring. A voice therapist can improve your public-speaking voice, but Throat Chakra balancing will improve your subtle communication skills, by drawing heart energies into your everyday speech.

For people such as monks who follow a specific spiritual path, these two chakras are where inner light forms, ready to be released through the voice as prayer, hymn, chant or song. This changes their relationship to the mundane world of matter, using the vibrational frequencies of pure spirit.

Throat imbalances are concerned with self-expression. Clearly we all need to speak our truth; this becomes easier once you overcome initial barriers of shyness or social or religious control. Because of the inherent strength of this chakra, a useful affirmation to make is along the lines of 'At every appropriate opportunity I will express my higher wisdom to others.'

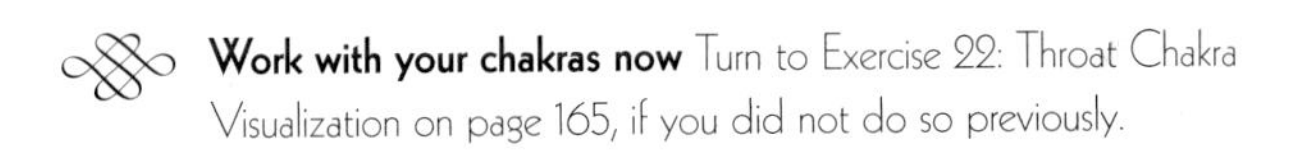

Work with your chakras now Turn to Exercise 22: Throat Chakra Visualization on page 165, if you did not do so previously.

Chakras and sound

Sound is commonly understood as a vibration that travels through a medium, usually air. However, sound also travels through water and blood, as well as through denser materials such as flesh and bone. The all-encompassing word 'sound', for these purposes, includes the speaking voice, singing voice and musical instruments.

Using the voice with or without accompanying instruments, I now want to introduce you to the benefits of mantras (including Bija mantras for the chakras), as well as to voice toning and overtoning. *You don't need to be a good singer to do this!*

Mantras

A mantra is repetitive vocalization of sacred words, syllables or prayer, using voice intonations. Used personally or ceremonially in a group, it produces altered states of consciousness by reducing brainwave levels. Profound realizations are achievable through pure concentrated focus of mind, body and spirit to connect with the core level of our Being.

Bija mantras

These are one-word mantras specific to the chakras, with their origins deep within ancient Hindu and Buddhist teachings. See page 156 for full details.

Voice toning

The express purpose of using the music in your voice for toning is to cause resonation within your physical body and/or etheric fields. Toning involves no melody, no words, no rhythm and no harmony – just the sound of the vibrating breath: re-sonance.

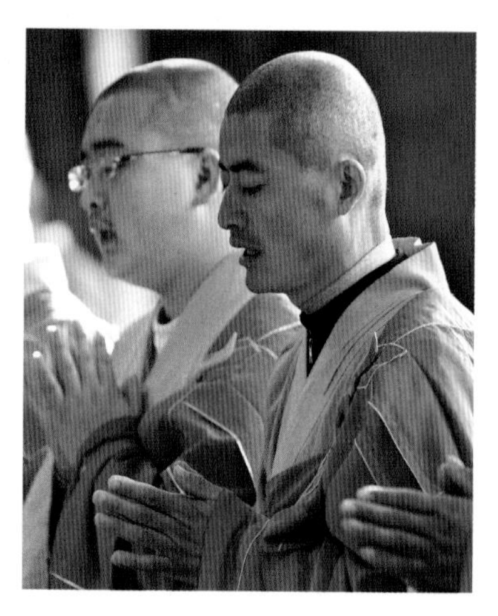

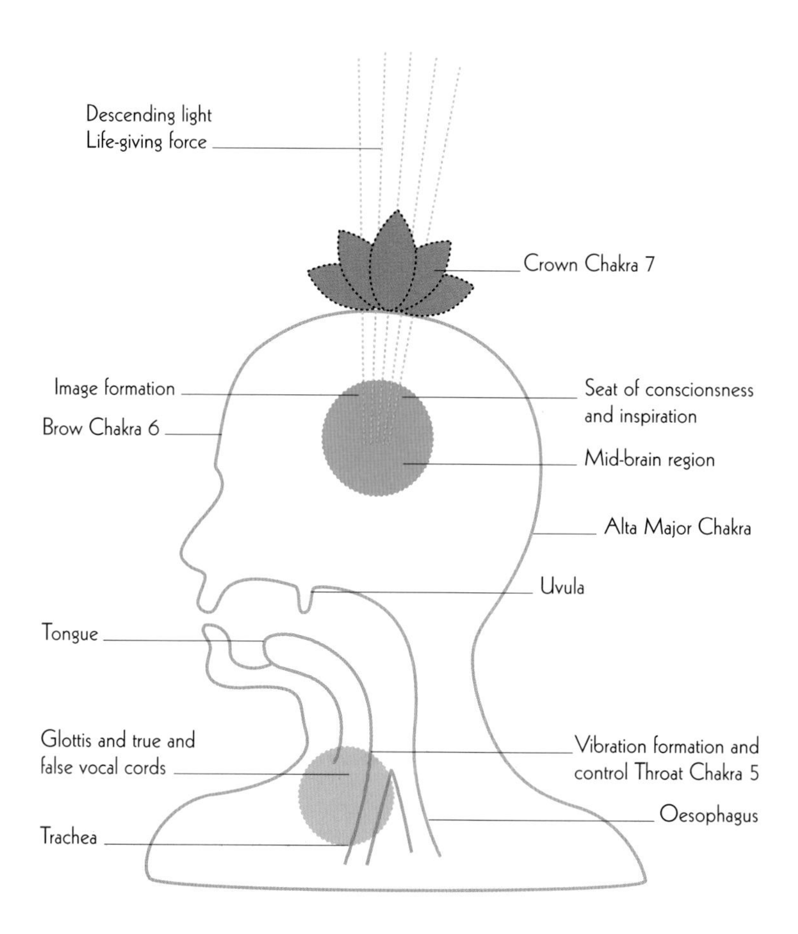

Voice toning can:

- Restore balance and harmony to your mind, emotions and body;
- Awaken and deepen your sense of self;
- Align you to the deepest vibration of soul and spirit;
- Synchronize your brainwaves and help relieve tension;
- Develop your voice–ear connection;
- Improve stamina and concentration;
- Expand your body's ability to breathe deeply.

On the path of toning, you move toward the source of your own inner balance, creativity, well-being and freedom.

When doing any of the sound exercises at the end of this section, begin by feeling calm and centred; drink a little pure water, blow your nose and clear your throat. Correct posture and breathing are important. Breath should be inhaled through the nostrils and out through the mouth – a steady breathing rhythm indicates that you are relaxed. Make your inhaled breath long, slow and as deep as possible. Do not allow your mind to wander or weaken, through thoughts such as 'I can't do it'. Instead, resonate with the frequency of what is forming within you. Enjoy the moment of bliss as you pause before releasing the sound; then focus on the chakra or place to which you wish the sound energy to go. When releasing the sound, do so as slowly as you can by allowing your tones to last for as long as possible. During inhalation, check your posture so that your lungs are fully but comfortably expanded, and each time try to breathe a little deeper and slower.

Keep repeating the appropriate sounds until you have focused your intention on each chakra. Always finish toning with grateful acceptance of what you have achieved at the physical, emotional, mental and spiritual levels. You will find suggestions concerning which tones to use on page 155.

Overtoning

In many references to the use of the voice for toning, mention is made of 'overtoning'. In Bija mantras, for example, you may discover a dot over the letter M; you may also see it written as 'ang' or 'ung' – the 'n' and/or the 'g' give the vital clue to expressing an overtone above the tone, and are an indicator that an overtone sound should be aimed for, by consciously strengthening the muscles surrounding the glottis in conjunction with the appropriate controlled release of breath. Simply begin by exploring different positions of the tongue, glottis and nasal passages while sounding the tone. Overtoning becomes a valuable exercise in muscle control and creates a magical effect, capable of relaxing you into deep alpha and theta brainwave levels. There is a whole beautiful world to explore if you are so inclined, but don't think you've failed if you are unable to produce 'overtones'.

Nada yoga: toning vowels

Nada yoga is the ancient yogic practice of using mantras and sounds in order to elevate consciousness. In ancient times, within Sanskrit, Hebrew and Chinese cultures, vowels were considered sacred. They are an expression of subtle energy. Consonants articulate that subtle energy into shapes. This is why vowels are toned for the chakra centres. To speak or tone the vowel sounds requires breath (ether) to pass out through an open mouth.

Try softly repeating the separate vowels A, E, I, O, U, and notice the effect this has upon you. Let go of any left-brain logical deductions as you do this exercise. As you learn to apply these vowels to the chakra centres, remember that it is always important to ascend through the chakras and then descend, so as to ground the energies. Ascending tones suggest movement toward the transcendence of matter into cosmic reality. Descending tones suggest movement from cosmic refinement into the denseness of matter.

There is a tremendous difference between listening to someone else toning or chanting and doing it yourself.

TONING VOWELS FOR THE CHAKRA CENTRES

CHAKRA (SANSKRIT NAME)	ELEMENT	KEYWORD	NOTE	VOWEL (AS IN)	CHAKRA (ENGLISH NAME)
Muladhara	Earth	Depth	Note of C	U (UH)	Base/Kanda
Svadisthana	Water	Flowing	Note of D	OO (TOO)	Sacral
Manipura	Fire	Opening	Note of E	O (GO)	Solar plexus
Anahata	Air	Fullness	Note of F	A (PA)	Heart
Vishuddha	Ether	Balance	Note of G	I (EYE)	Throat
Ajna	Mind	Intensity	Note of A	A (AYE)	Third Eye
Sahasrara	Pure consciousness	Wisdom	Note of B	E (EEE)	Crown

Nada yoga: Bija mantras

Through the use of Bija mantras – one-word mantras specific to the chakras – the chakra system is brought alive. Traditionally they are intoned silently, although since sound is an all-over body experience, you may like to vocalize them out loud using the following scale. Remember to breathe correctly and deeply, so that the sound resonates within your whole body. With focused consciousness and by learning through practice, you will increase your overall state of wellness.

Bija literally means 'seed'. Through intention, correct breathing and vocalization, the seed will germinate and flourish within your awareness as well as in your physical body.

Repeated use of the Bija mantras creates the possibility of transformation, simply because vibration directed with powerfully focused intention aligns the body's physical structure at a molecular level. An Indian 'mala' or 108-bead necklace is used as a method of

THE SAPTAK SCALE AND ASSOCIATED BIJA MANTRAS

SAPTAK SCALE	NATURE SOUND	DIATONIC SCALE	CHAKRA	BIJA MANTRA/ OVERTONE SYMBOL (G)
Sadja/Sa	Peacock's cry	C	Muladhara/Base/Kanda	LAM(g)
Risabha/Re	Cow calling her calf	D	Svadisthana/Sacral	VAM(g)
Gandhara/Ga	Goat bleating	E	Manipura/Navel	RAM(g)
Madhyama/Ma	Heron's cry	F#	Anahata/Heart	YAM(g)
Panchame/Pa	Cuckoo's song	G	Vishuddha/Throat	HAM(g)
Dhaivata/Da	Horse's neigh	A	Ajna/Third Eye	OM(g)
Nishada/Ni	Elephant trumpeting	B ♭	Sahasrara/Crown	OM(g)

counting the repetitions, so that the mind can concentrate upon the mantras.

The seven notes of the Indian musical scale associated with Bija mantras, called the Saptak, were established in India by the 2nd century BCE and related humans to the sounds of Nature. The Western musical scale below is only an approximation of this Saptak scale. All traditional mantras are internalized in five stages:

- Likhita: through writing;
- Vaikhari: through speaking and sounding;
- Upamshu: through whispering;
- Manasa: through thinking;
- Ajapa: through uninterrupted inner repetition.

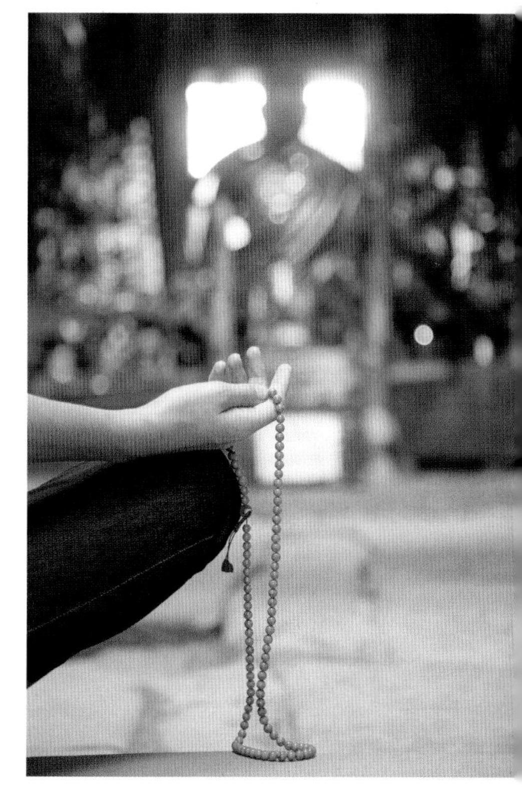

Work with your chakras now Turn to Exercise 23: Sound Experience on page 168.

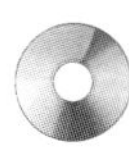

Work with the CD now Play CD reference Track 4, to hear the same Sound Experience.

Energy Medicine

Energy Medicine (sometimes called Vibrational Healing) is a wide-ranging, diverse, holistic type of healthcare and healing that provides treatment by balancing the human energy system. Most importantly, Energy Medicine harmonizes with the natural healing abilities of the body, because it has an innate drive to function at its highest possible state of health. Dis-ease (deliberately hyphenated) is your body demonstrating that you need to start listening to it because something is out of balance.

While doctors are excellent at treating emergencies, they are not so adept at treating dis-ease. Simply addressing the symptoms does not usually get to the original energetic cause. Often symptoms are masked by prescribed drugs, and the imbalance will continue. However, in serious conditions, always heed your doctor's advice.

In many instances Energy Medicine, which focuses upon the chakras, will enable a return to a state of wellness and ease. This is aided by slowing down and, most importantly, learning how to relax and taking numerous stops along the way, to restore optimum balance by developing a harmonious relationship within ourselves.

Scientific discoveries show that our energy system (chakras, meridians, subtle-energy field, and so on) vibrates at many subtle levels. Usually it lies beyond the point where most people can hear or perceive it, but with some practice it can be sensed by any dedicated person.

A healer or practitioner in Energy Medicine uses finely tuned energy-sensing skills to assess and then balance the subtle-energy system, aiming to access and guide a person's subtle energy and assist in its transformation; sometimes it needs to be increased, and at other times decreased. A healer will use crystals, sound, light, colour and numerous other methods, or will channel healing energy through their hands. This workshop-in-a-book enables you to develop these skills to use upon yourself.

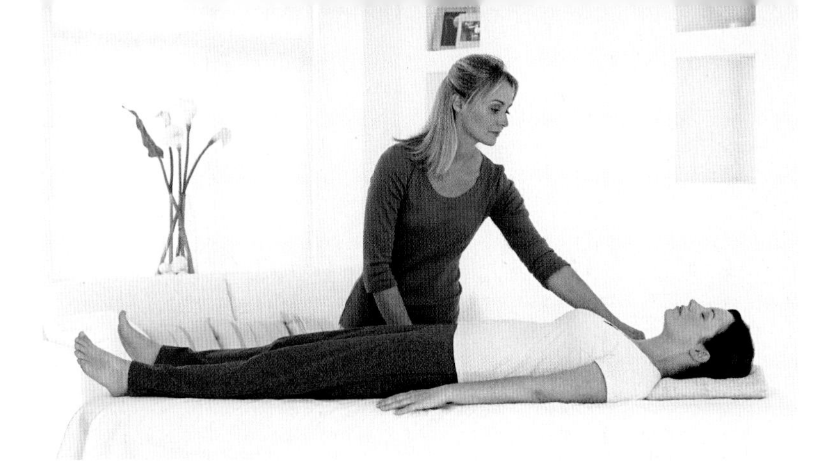

How does it work?

Physicists tell us that everything is simply energy. Energy has a range of low to high frequencies. Lower frequencies are more dense, so they are the ones we can see in our physical world – everything from our pet cat to the table at which we sit. Higher frequencies are much less dense – they are the subtle energies that we refer to when we talk of auras and chakras. Physicists describe how energies interpenetrate one another, from the microscopic cellular and DNA level to the movement of planets and stars in the cosmos.

As we have already discussed, the seven main chakras are specialized energy centres working to regulate the flow of pranic life-force within the body. It enters the body field at a chakra and travels through the network of nadis to particular cells, organs and tissues. These reciprocate by resonating with that chakra's unique frequency. This subtle-energy system is complementary to physical body systems such as the nervous, digestive and circulatory systems. When we interact *consciously* with the energy system, we get to the root cause of dis-ease.

The adverse effects of EMF and noise

This book would be incomplete without mentioning the potential effects upon our chakras of the external electromagnetic fields (EMFs) that we are subjected to in our daily lives. Domestic electrical appliances give out a measurable force field, which may particularly affect the Base and Sacral Chakras if we are exposed to the source for a continuous length of time. So check to ensure that these electrical force fields (and the pulsed micro-waves from cellphones, TVs and other electrical units) are at a safe distance from where you and your family sleep. Any EMF force fields near the head are particularly dangerous to the higher chakras.

Noise is legally defined as a pollutant in a number of countries. Medical studies confirm the adverse effects of noise on the hearing, heart rate, blood pressure, sleep and mental health, as well as on physical performance, measured by inappropriate levels of adrenaline, nor-adrenaline and melatonin, which have implications for chakra energies.

The effect of sound upon an unborn child in a mother's womb is particularly important. The pineal centre appears at the fifth week in the developing human embryo. By the 18th week the sense of hearing has become active, and its first function is to give 'food' to the brain. It is wise to protect your unborn child from excessively loud noise and music by placing a cushion over your lower chakra areas, because metaphysical teachings regard the foetus's chakras and subtle-energy system as the 'template' upon which life builds from the moment of conception.

For the first seven years of a child's life close contact with the mother is vital, to ensure that the child's etheric body maintains vital interdependence with its mother's energies. Therefore a mother's attention to maintaining wellness through chakra balancing also has implications for the child.

The adverse effects of chemicals

A whole range of chemical vibrational frequencies severely affects chakra functioning. So examine the many ways in which you can bring your life more into tune with Nature, challenging dis-ease and balancing your chakras. Try to choose natural fibres for clothing and bedding, such as cotton, hemp, wool, silk or linen, because they permit the healthy functioning of the auric field. Avoid chemicals and additives in your food – stay natural and read the labels. Especially avoid chemical cleaners such as bleach; a natural alternative for all home cleaning applications is vinegar.

Optional advanced exercise Turn to Exercise 25: Cutting Emotional 'Cords' on page 174 for an optional advanced exercise.

THROAT CHAKRA EXERCISES

The following exercises develop the Throat Chakra or Vishuddha, which expresses where you are on your path of life through speech, song or devotional words such as hymns, mantras and chants. It reflects how you treat others and whether you speak your truth. You will learn how to rebalance it by practising 'Bija mantras' with the help of the CD, as well as other more advanced methods.

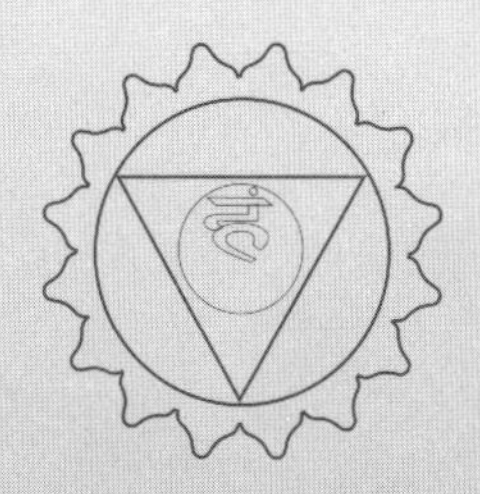

Developing intuition

Do this exercise before reading beyond this page. It will become a record of your Throat Chakra – showing your ability to express yourself – to which you can refer back in order to chart your progress.

Exercise 21 SENSING AND DRAWING MY THROAT CHAKRA

You will need: a set of coloured pencils or pens (all colours, including magenta); keep the book open, ready to colour in the body outline opposite, which represents you (sign and date it before you begin).

- **To begin,** take five minutes sitting in a quiet place, breathing slowly, relaxing and closing your eyes. Now start to sense your body and your aura. Release any emotions that arise. Forget anything you have ever heard or read about chakras and auras. You are simply 'sensing' how your own unique energies are flowing at present. Check from your feet up to your head to pick up any little clues that your body is giving you. Sense your auric energy field around you as well. Now focus upon your Throat Chakra area. What is it 'telling' you? What can you sense? Does it feel free, flowing, harmonious? Or is an old pain or trauma held there? Does this area feel fluid and open – or have you shut off all feelings and thoughts of this chakra?
- **When you feel ready,** open your eyes and – immediately and without thinking – quickly colour in the Throat Chakra area and any other parts of the body (and the surrounding page) as you wish. There is no right or wrong place to apply the colour: it is entirely up to you.
- **Read the interpretation** on page 164 after completing this exercise.

My sensing and drawing my throat chakra experience

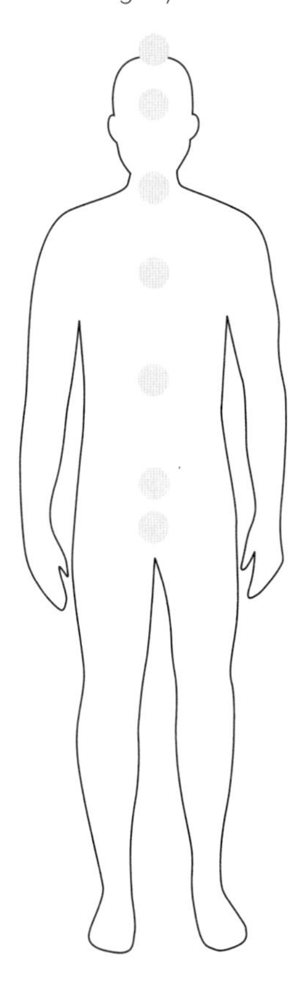

Date ______________________ Signature ______________________

Assessing my results for Exercise 21

A balanced Throat Chakra will show strong and vibrant colours of turquoise, blue or green. It will reflect your inner will, self-expression and ability to communicate in a caring way. It may also reflect the ability to speak your own truth without hurting others, and a developed singing skill.

An unbalanced Throat Chakra will show either very weak or very strong colours. These colours may be dark shades – black, brown or grey or a strong, dull red. When weakened, it will reflect depression, dependence and an inability to express yourself. Overactivity may make you overreactive, intolerant and hurtful to others, especially in an uncaring choice of words. Frustration held in the Throat Chakra may manifest as strong anger or violence.

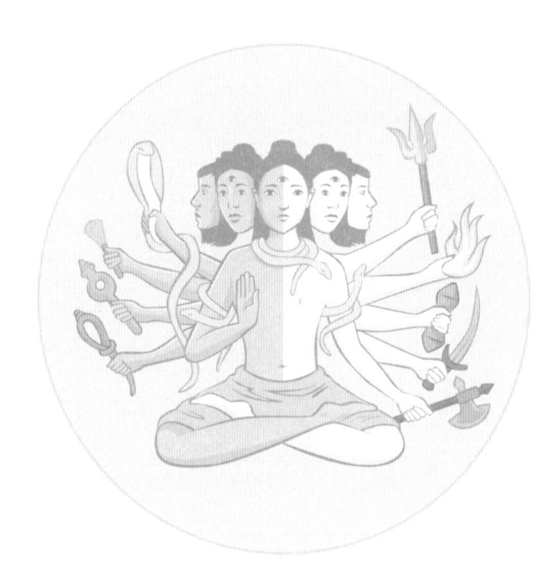

Meditative visualization

This visualization exercise will increase your energy, help to lift depression and boost your immune system. Ideally it should be done outside, while lying on your back looking up at a pure blue sky. If this is not possible, make yourself comfortable inside and imagine that you are gazing into the sky.

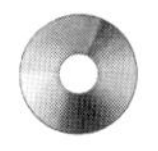

Exercise 22 THROAT CHAKRA VISUALIZATION

CD REFERENCE TRACK 2 (OPTIONAL) (TO FOLLOW THE SCRIPT, TURN TO PAGE 110)

- **To begin,** do Exercise 15: Complete Relaxation on page 110, using CD reference Track 2 (optional).
- **Then visualize a pure sky-blue colour** all around you. Imagine you are gazing across a very calm sea that merges with the sky into a shimmering pale turquoise in the far distance.
- **Feel that you can breathe in** pure sky-blue colour into your body. Imagine that you are immersed in a sea of tranquillity and can hear the sounds of the sea blending with the rhythmic sounds of your own body.
- **Know that this colour cleanses** and refreshes your physical body. It brings a spiritual dimension to your whole energy field and chakras. It especially boosts your energy levels by clearing unwanted elements from your Throat Chakra region.
- **Now imagine a bridge of Light** spanning the sea, which it is possible to cross. On arriving at the other side, you meet a beautiful glowing 'Light being'. It may be your guardian angel or Archangel Michael, who brings the qualities of communication and self-expression. Whoever it is, allow them to place their healing hands upon you and transmit Light throughout your whole mind/body/spirit complex.

- **Feel the warmth** from the Light being's hands removing any pain or disharmony from your body. Feel their hands removing any stress and tension from your mind. See them dispersing into the vast Ocean of Life. When they have finished their healing work, they remove their hands, but the warmth and sense of well-being remains with you.
- **Realize that we are each a tiny drop** in the vast Ocean of Life, but as each drop is important in the great universal plan, so you too are unique and important.
- **Thank the Light being** and return the way you came, across the bridge of Light.
- **On reaching your starting point again,** breathe in pure sky-blue colour, reconnect with your physical body, and finally open your eyes.
- **Now consider** the questions on page 167.

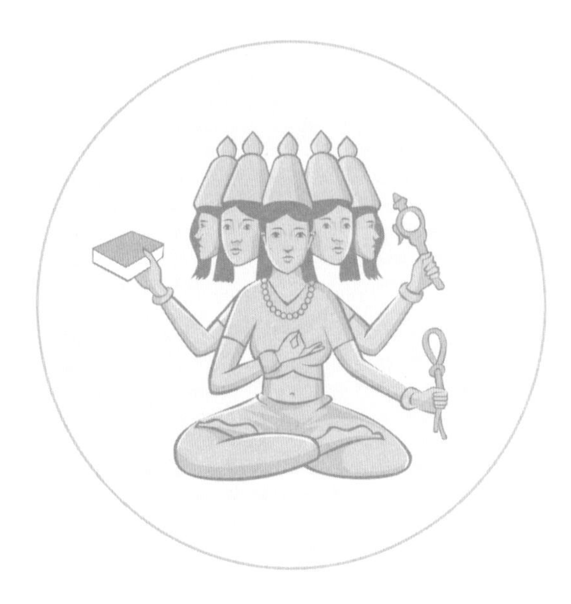

My throat chakra visualization experience

Date ______________________________

Where I did my visualization ______________________________

____

____

____

____

What I experienced ______________________________

____

____

____

____

What I can learn from this visualization ______________________________

____

____

____

____

Sounding the Bija mantras

This Sound Experience exercise introduces you to sounding the Bija mantras (see page 156). As a regular practice it is helpful to repeat the Bija mantra at least three times with each chakra. Sit comfortably on cushion or upright chair. Ensure you will not be interrupted. It is best not to have eaten for at least an hour, but do have water to hand. Begin with lighting a candle.

Toning the Bija mantras is not a diagnostic tool; it is about creating transformation so avoid any expectations during toning. Don't be surprised, or think you have failed, if you have sensed nothing – sometimes seeds take time to germinate! Repeat the exercise as many times as you can manage, simply enjoy being a human being instead of a human doing.

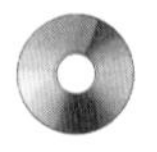

Exercise 23 SOUND EXPERIENCE

CD REFERENCE TRACK 4 (TO FOLLOW THE SCRIPT, SEE BELOW)

- **To begin,** relax your shoulders, keeping your spine straight. Clear your nose and throat. Sit in an upright position, with your palms facing upward and your index fingers touching the thumbs (this is called the 'Chin or Jnana Mudra').
- **Focus on the candle flame,** the rhythms of your heart and breathing.
- **Remain silently focused** for a minute, carefully avoiding any external thought intrusion.
- **Place your left hand** on the perineum (the region surrounding the urogenital and anal openings) for the Base Chakra (if you wish) and focus on your Base Chakra.
- * **Draw a full breath into your lungs,** continuing to concentrate and letting your voice make a sound expressing the Bija LAM (sounds like 'laarmm').
- **Allow your lungs to empty slowly** while maintaining your inner focus.

- **Then begin to focus on the next chakra**, placing your left hand (if you so wish) below the navel.
- **Repeat from * above**, but with the Bija VAM (sounds like 'vaarmm').
- **Repeat from * above**, placing your hand on your solar plexus, sounding the Bija RAM (sounds like 'raarmm').
- **Repeat from * above**, placing your hand on heart, sounding the Bija YAM (sounds like 'yaarmm').
- **Repeat from * above**, placing your hand on the throat, sounding the Bija HAM (sounds like 'haarmm').
- **Repeat from * above**, placing your hand on the forehead, sounding the Bija OM (sounds like 'aumm').
- **Repeat from * above**, placing the palm of your hand downward on top of your head, sounding the Bija OM (sounds like 'aumm').
- **Finish by breathing slowly** and deeply, allowing anything that you wish to release to pass from you with each exhalation.
- **Give silent thanks** for this precious time that you have been able to keep with yourself.
- **Record any notes** that you wish to make on pages 170–71.

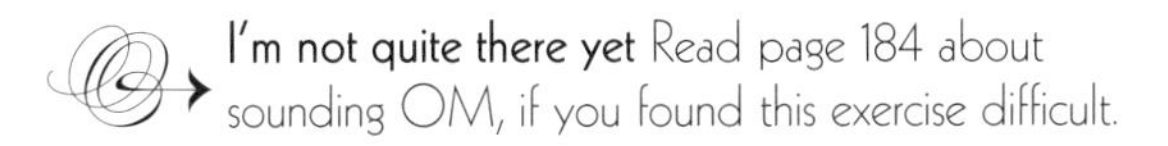

I'm not quite there yet Read page 184 about sounding OM, if you found this exercise difficult.

My sound experience

Date ______________________________

- What, if anything, did I experience at a physical, emotional, mental and spiritual level when I toned LAM? ______________________________

- What, if anything, did I experience at a physical, emotional, mental and spiritual level when I toned VAM? ______________________________

- What, if anything, did I experience at a physical, emotional, mental and spiritual level when I toned RAM? ______________________________

- What, if anything, did I experience at a physical, emotional, mental and spiritual level when I toned YAM?

- What, if anything, did I experience at a physical, emotional, mental and spiritual level when I toned HAM?

- What, if anything, did I experience at a physical, emotional, mental and spiritual level when I toned OM (for the Third Eye)?

- What, if anything, did I experience at a physical, emotional, mental and spiritual level when I toned OM (for the Crown)?

Recharging the Throat Chakra

For this exercise you need to be in a place where you will not be disturbed for approximately half an hour – indoors is okay, but it would be even better to be sitting outside. Wherever you choose, your spine must be as straight as possible and your chin pulled in, to straighten the back of your neck.

Choose two cleansed and dedicated small pieces of natural turquoise (if you choose to use crystals) and hold one in each hand. Place 'grounding' stones, such as heavy beach pebbles under your feet (see page 27 for more about 'grounding' stones). Light a special candle if you wish.

Exercise 24 COLOUR-BREATHING WITH CRYSTALS

CD REFERENCE TRACK 2 (OPTIONAL) (TO FOLLOW THE SCRIPT, SEE PAGE 110)

- **To begin,** sit in an upright chair or a cross-legged yoga posture. Ensure that you are fully relaxed.
- **Close your eyes** and breathe slowly, visualizing your incoming breath as a clear, bright turquoise-blue light. Breathe deeply for a few minutes, focusing on the Throat Chakra. Feel this coloured breath suffusing the area of your physical throat and neck and its chakra with energy.
- **Now feel this coloured light** spreading across your shoulders, balancing the minor chakras there.
- **'Wrap' a cloak of turquoise light** around your whole body and auric field for protection.
- **Return to normal breathing** and, when you feel ready, slowly open your eyes.
- **Now consider** the questions on page 173.

My colour-breathing with crystals experience

Date ______________________________

How well did I relax? Well / It was difficult / I couldn't relax at all

Did the colour-breathing help me to focus on my Throat Chakra?
Yes / No / A bit, but then I lost the focus / Don't know

How did this exercise affect me? ______________________________

Does my Throat Chakra feel more balanced? Yes / No / A bit / Don't know

Releasing emotional suffering

Today, in an advanced exercise, you are going to release – cut the 'cords' – that tie you to outdated emotional suffering. You will cut them *once only* and it will be *for ever*. This is a symbolic act and 'rite of passage'. You will be calling upon the Force of Grace, which, if invoked by your superconsciousness (your higher self), cannot fail to respond.

Ideally you should be outside in a quiet, natural place; alternatively place a chair before an open window. This release is most powerful when done in the presence of two friends: one to witness, the other (the 'reader') to read the words, slowly, for you to repeat. However, it can be done on your own, but the words *must always be read slowly out loud* and with conviction. You do not need to tell your friends any details of the emotional suffering that you are about to release – in fact, it is much better not to transfer any of it to them. So don't chat; just make time and space for this special act.

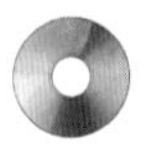

Exercise 25 CUTTING EMOTIONAL 'CORDS'

CD REFERENCE TRACK 2 (OPTIONAL) (TO FOLLOW THE SCRIPT, TURN TO PAGE 110)

- **To begin,** play CD Track 2 (optional) to ensure that you are fully relaxed, then sit up.
- **Get your friends to stand** one on each side of you and slightly behind you. (The release that liberates you from emotional 'cords' works through your physical, emotional, mental and spiritual bodies; it is cathartic, so you don't want someone standing in front of you to take on any negativity.)
- **The 'reader' begins,** saying the following words, line by line, which you then speak clearly out loud:

Superconsciousness, by the Force of Grace,
I formally rescind all ties and attachments
to outdated emotional suffering
entered into in this or any other lifetime.
I cut these 'cords' that have bound and limited me
And replace them with light that suffuses my
Energy body with joy.
May the power of that release
be fully manifest in my consciousness. [deep, releasing out-breath]
And so it is.

- **Now record** your experience on page 176.
- **Note** 'Energy Medicine' such as this does not normally conflict with medication, although those with mental health issues should consult their healthcare provider.

Later, when you feel ready to do so, you may also work on the Throat Chakra with any of the other balancing methods mentioned on other pages of this book. Consult the chart on page 147 to ascertain which aromatherapy oil to use, which yoga postures, colour breathing, and so on.

My cutting emotional 'cords' experience

Date of release of emotional suffering ________________________________

Do not discuss what you experienced with those friends who helped you. Instead, write below any positive thoughts or feelings that you wish to record. ________________

Use a separate piece of paper to draw anything positive that you experienced (optional)

Should you have experienced any negative emotions, use a separate piece of paper to write them down or draw them and burn it immediately.

Remember that this is a once-only release of energy. It does not need to be repeated. If, at some future date, your mind begins to dwell on similar emotional issues, look back to this day, remember that you released all past and future emotional suffering, congratulate yourself and celebrate.

THE THIRD EYE CHAKRA: AJNA

Work with your chakras now Before you read further, turn to Exercise 26: Sensing and Drawing my Third Eye Chakra on page 194.

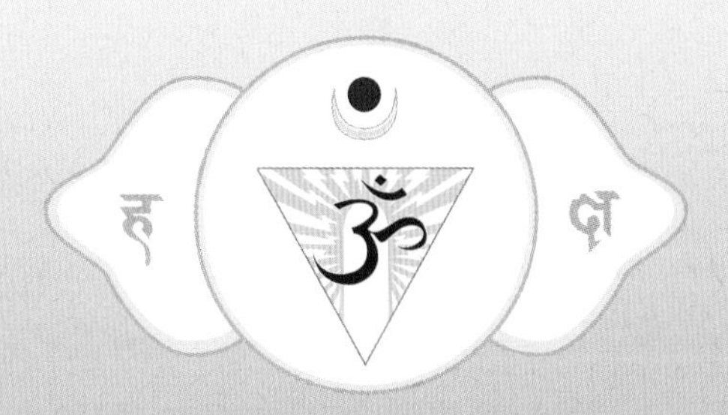

About my Third Eye Chakra

Keypoints: Resonates with the subtle element of Spirit and the colour deep blue; concerned with extra-sensory perception (ESP), clarity, intuition (inner teaching) and balancing our higher and lower selves.

The sixth chakra, the Third Eye or Brow Chakra, is the centre where we control the power of our mind. The Sanskrit name, *Ajna*, means 'to know' or 'to command' and it is traditionally regarded as the place where conflict takes place between ego and Spirit. It is also where we can release the limitations imposed upon us by the psychological construct of ego, which by rights should have already been dealt with at the Solar Plexus Chakra. Once this is achieved, we become open to 'inner sight' through the symbolic celestial marriage of sun and moon, mind and body.

This chakra is depicted with two petals in indigo or white, bearing Sanskrit letters. These petals symbolize the right and left sides of the brain, and represent the combination of the two polarities of human existence. The left side of the brain is our rational, analytical side, while the right is our intuitive, creative and experiential side. Traditionally a downward-pointing triangle is shown at Ajna, signifying the importance of integrating masculine and feminine energies at this stage of human spiritual evolution. This means that we will each become complete within ourselves, no longer depending upon others for our security or nurture. In fact the goddess of Ajna, Shakti Hakini, also illustrates this point, because her many minds are divinely pure – achieved by drinking the divine 'nectar' that constantly flows toward the Base Chakra.

All the ancient texts recommend 'awakening' the Third Eye Chakra slowly. Deep-blue light stimulates this chakra, which is sometimes symbolized by a blue sapphire.

Optional advanced exercise Turn to Exercise 27: Candle Meditation on page 197, to deepen your experience of meditation using a candle.

CHART OF THE THIRD EYE CHAKRA

Colour of influence	Blue
Complementary light colour	Orange
Colour to calm	Blue and pale blue
Physical location	Centre of brow
Physiological system	Endocrine and nervous systems
Endocrine system	Pituitary
Key issues	Balancing higher and lower self and trusting inner guidance
Inner teaching	Completing and clearing karmic lessons
Energy action	Merging masculine and feminine energies
Balancing crystals	Lapis lazuli and any deep-blue crystal
Balancing aromatherapy oils	Frankincense, basil (in moderation)
Balancing herbal teas	Juniper/lemon balm/chamomile, or a mix (for the brain) of ginkgo, peppermint, nettle, rosehip, basil and anise
Balancing yoga position (*asana*)	Adho Mukha Avanasana (dog face down), yoga mudra in Padmasana (advanced pose), Halasana (Plough), Matsyasana (Fish).
Mantra/tone	OM in the note of A
Helpful musical instruments/music	Harp
Planet/astrological sign/natural House	Uranus/Saturn/Aquarius/Capricorn/eleventh: objectives/tenth: protection
Reiki hand position	Palms covering the face, then lift off to sides of head on the temples
Power animal (Native American tradition)	Spirit guides and ancestors

Body/Third Eye Chakra connections

This chakra's action on the body's glandular system occurs through the pituitary gland, which lies behind the eyes and is known as the 'leader of the endocrine orchestra'. Our physiological balance and growth are maintained and monitored by the pituitary gland. It is more active at puberty and is concerned with female fertility and pregnancy. The physical location of the Third Eye Chakra is in the centre of the brow, just above the eyebrows, and it is related to the brain, eyes, ears, nose and nervous system.

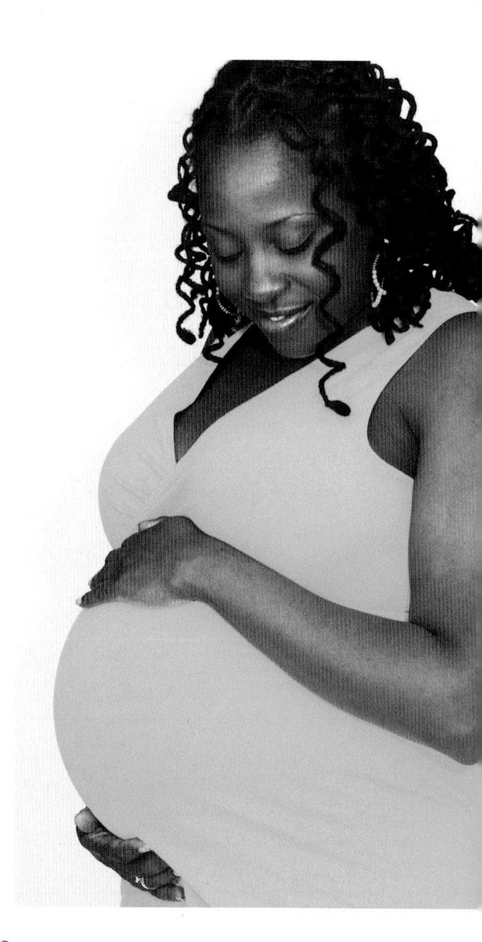

When this chakra is imbalanced you may experience headaches, migraines, eye and sinus problems, catarrh, hayfever and hormonal fluctuations. Sleeplessness and disturbing dreams may be encountered if you overstimulate this chakra. Relaxation is key to its balance, coupled with many types of 'Energy Medicine' (which was introduced on page 158).

Ajna is particularly receptive to Energy Medicine in the form of visualization, meditation, crystals, colour, coloured light, essential oils and the high vibration of flower essences. You may awaken this chakra by tapping it a number of times with the middle finger of your right hand, then massaging it with a circular clockwise movement. Visualize your Third Eye Chakra – your inner eye, the 'Eye of Shiva' – being cleaned, cleared and balanced.

Associated chakras

The Third Eye Chakra is connected to a smaller chakra called the Soma Chakra, meaning nectar or 'amrita'. This is depicted as a lotus with 12 petals with a silver crescent moon at the centre, said to be the source of the nectar. It is positioned at the centre of the hairline. Lavender-blue light stimulates this chakra. Tantric yoga describes how priests traditionally maintained celibacy to transmute their sexual energies in the Soma Chakra in order to gain enlightenment. It is considered to contain the combined energies of the godhead: Brahma the creator, Vishnu the preserver and Shiva the destroyer.

Two other minor paired chakras are also associated with the Third Eye, and particularly with developing healing abilities; they are the small Temple Chakras at either side of our head.

“All strength, all healing of every nature is the changing of the vibrations from within – the attuning of the Divine within the living tissue of a body to creative energies. This alone is healing.”
Edgar Cayce, American healer and visionary

Work with your chakras now Turn to Exercise 30: Colour-Breathing for my Third Eye Chakra on page 206.

Third Eye energy and imbalances

Energetically this chakra helps us to understand the world around us intellectually, honing our ability to accurately remember the past and helping us to envision the future, while remaining firmly anchored in the present *now* moment. The Third Eye, our inner perceptive faculty, opens our physical eyes to the beauty of the natural world that is all around us, if we take the trouble to look – even if we live in a city. This chakra, in its own way, energetically 'channels' beauty, art and positive vision as vital soul 'food'. It shows us the beauty in others, and in the simplest things in life.

If it is energetically blocked, the Third Eye may make us over-intellectualize, become egotistical or deluded, suffer from memory loss, show paranoia, negativity or deeply engrained sarcasm, or be drawn into controlling types of religion or causes such as conspiracy theories. We might come across to others as controlling perfectionists, putting on a mask for the sake of appearances, instead of displaying honest self-expression.

Physical manifestations

Physiologically, migraine headaches may result from a reduced supply of oxygen to the brain (although they can be food-related). From a body/mind perspective, migraines suggest that deeply held needs are being thwarted. Sometimes they are caused by an overload of responsibility that denies fulfilment in a given area. Look at your lifestyle choices, and whether you need to look deeper into your soul through your inner eye.

Do you have frequent headaches, sinus/ear problems or endocrine imbalances? At an energetic level, this is caused by not wanting to see or hear something that is important to your inner growth and soul's journey. One suggestion to remedy this is to follow the proverb 'Do not put off until tomorrow something that can be done today.' Working with visualization exercises, particularly on the Third Eye, will help to open up new possibilities for you that, if absorbed at deep inner levels, may improve your well-being.

A stiff neck may indicate that you are limiting yourself by only wanting to look in one direction. Work on the Throat and Third Eye Chakras, together with the Base Chakra, to give yourself increased energy levels and to repattern the effects of limitation.

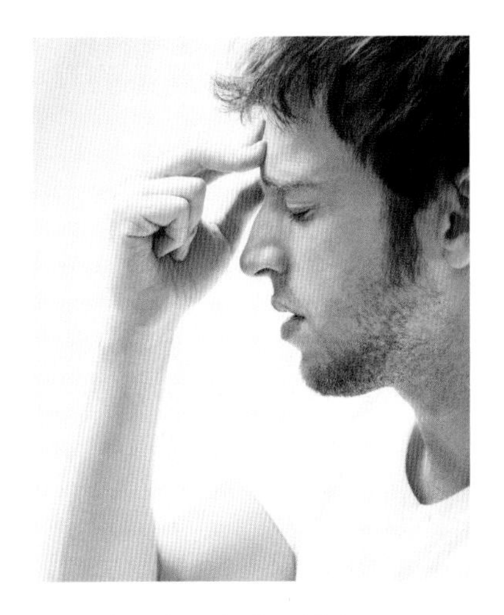

Balancing the whole chakra system – together with focus upon the Heart (self-worth), Throat (self-expression) and Third Eye (Brow) Chakras (visualization of a goal) – will help many symptoms of dis-ease. Chakra balancing through the methods described in this workshop-in-a-book generally brings peaceful acceptance of physical ailments, which may sometimes be ameliorated by adjusting the energy flow through appropriate chakras. Do remember, though, that this is a type of Energy Medicine that is primarily intended to balance energy. The effects are sometimes immediately beneficial to the physical body, but sometimes a 'healing crisis' results, which releases long-held, deeply entrenched dis-ease. If this occurs, know that the body, in its wisdom, is using its own method to restore equilibrium.

Work with your chakras now Turn to Exercise 29: Dowsing the Third Eye on page 203, to check the balance of your Third Eye with a pendulum.

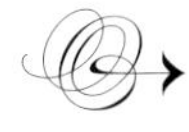

I'm not quite there yet. Turn to Exercise 28: Releasing Negative Patterns on page 199.

The sacred OM/AUM

OM/AUM is an ancient Sanskrit word, thought to be the primordial creative sound from which the universe and all of Creation first manifested. Originally it was set forth as the object of profound religious meditation, with the highest spiritual efficacy being attributed not only to the whole word, but also to the three sounds within it.

The two written words OM and AUM describe the same sound. A-U-M represents divine energy (Shakti) and unites the major trinity of Hindu gods: Brahma, Vishnu and Shiva in their three elementary aspects: Brahma Shakti (creation), Vishnu Shakti (preservation) and Shiva Shakti (liberation and/or destruction).

Going deeper in the act of voicing OM/AUM, we find that it consists of three phonemes (units of sound): a, u and m. It symbolizes the Three Vedas, the Hindu Trimurti or the three stages of birth, life and death respectively.

In Tibetan Buddhist tradition, OM ('AUM') represents different aspects of the trinity of the Body (A), Speech (U) and Mind (M) of the Buddha, or an enlightened being. Sounding the AUM in this manner puts one in resonance with these qualities of consciousness. Yet another esoteric teaching of OM ('AUM') reminds us that the 'A' represents the physical plane, the 'U' the mental and astral planes and the 'M' all that is beyond the reach of the intellect. OM ('AUM') is the initial syllable at the commencement of many mantras.

Mantrically repeating OM/AUM will help you connect with the still point within, which may be described as the 'Source' of who you really are. OM is not just a sound or vibration; it is not just a symbol. It enables us to touch the entire cosmos – whatever we can see, touch, hear and feel. It is all that is within our perception and all that is beyond our perception. It is the core of our very existence. If you think of OM only as a sound, a technique or a symbol of the divine, you will miss a profound opportunity to change your whole life and understand who you really are.

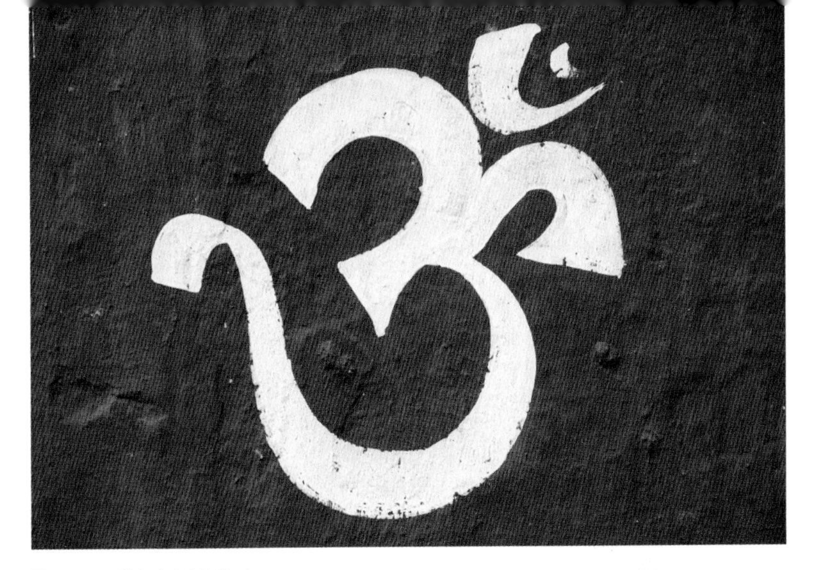

Toning OM/AUM

OM/AUM may be repeatedly toned as a mantra, but to achieve a path of deeper realization requires preparation. The following are guidelines for the beginner:

- Prepare to spend time somewhere you can be quiet and uninterrupted.
- Sit comfortably in an upright chair or in an appropriate yoga position.
- Become aware of your gentle, relaxed breathing.
- Reflect upon the meaning of OM/AUM and integrate these thoughts with your intention to sound the sacred word.
- *Breathe in deeply and, as you do so, visualize a fine strand of light entering through your Crown Chakra from somewhere way above. Feel that connection to the Light in your pineal gland/Crown Chakra area as you form a sound.
- Open your mouth, gently and slowly releasing your breath as you utter in equal length of time A... U... M..., taking care to pronounce the letters clearly and softly. (Enhance your facial muscular movements and give equal weight to each letter.)
- Take care not to force, strain or create tension.
- Enjoy the space after the out-breath and then repeat from *.
- Continue for a minimum of 5 to 10 minutes. When you have finished, be still, and in the silence absorb the vibration and, in turn, the deep realization of what you have created.

Using a crystal on my Third Eye

Having trained as a crystal healer, I recommend that you only *activate* the Third Eye Chakra with a crystal if you:

- Have already worked extensively with the chakras beneath it;
- Are prepared for a deep awakening;
- Are willing to enter other dimensional realities.

If so, use a cleansed clear quartz that is dedicated to your inner spiritual growth. Lie down and place the quartz on your brow for no more than ten minutes on the first occasion.

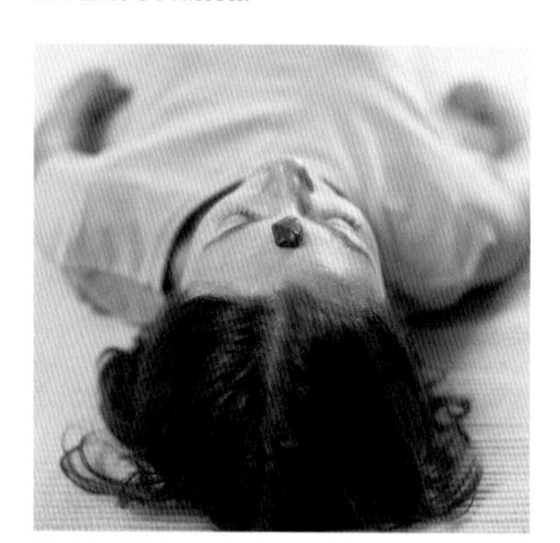

Other Third Eye actions

If you wish to *balance* the Third Eye Chakra, then ideally use lapis lazuli – a deep-blue stone with little golden veins in it – again for no more than ten minutes on the first occasion.

If you wish to *calm* the Third Eye Chakra, then ideally use emerald or sapphire. Although these may sound like expensive precious stones, they can be obtained very cheaply as uncut stones. Again use them for no more than ten minutes on the first occasion.

As you become more used to working with crystals, you can tape a small piece of emerald or sapphire to your Third Eye Chakra before you go to sleep, in order to have a calm night's sleep, untroubled by disturbing dreams. It may cause you to have wonderfully vivid and helpful dreams instead!

Making solarized water

Every chakra takes on and resonates with a specific energetic colour of light. It is a kind of 'food', which the chakra is drawing into the physical body as though it is liquid being poured through a funnel.

In this book, for ease of visualization, the predominant chakra colour is given, although these colours are never static or solely one shade of colour, because healers realize that there is continual movement in the energy body. Those who can see auric fields and chakras refer to the colours as swirling mist in constant motion. Detection work on the condition of auric fields and chakras can often lead to a perception of dis-ease before it manifests in the body.

Colour healers develop the ability to channel a specific colour or to use instruments to give coloured light. There is also a simple colour-healing vehicle called 'solarized water', which passes sunshine through high-quality translucent coloured glass into water, and this can easily be prepared at home. It should be made with pure

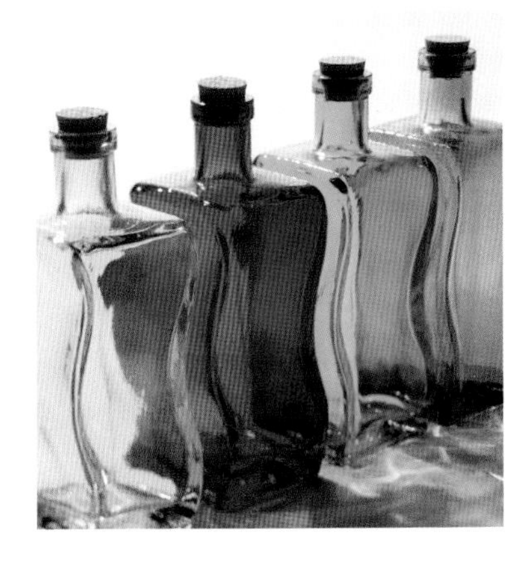

spring water, because water has the ability to take on different energetic encodings.

Select small, clean glass bottles or containers in a range of vibrant single colours (of course you may choose the appropriate chakra colour). Add the water and leave in the sun or strong daylight for up to 12 hours. The resulting coloured solarized water should be sipped slowly throughout the day between meals. This is a type of Energy Medicine that gives you a particular frequency of light-encoded water.

The meaning of colours

Different colours have different meanings when it comes to balancing the chakras.

Red ranges from very deep to a very pale red and has the slowest, longest wavelength of any colour. It is a powerful energizer and stimulant. Red increases blood supply to an area and improves circulation, of both physical and subtle energies. It should not be used where there is anger, anxiety or emotional issues.

Orange is more gentle in action than red and lies midway between the red and the yellow rays, therefore influencing physical vitality and intellect. Orange brings about changes in our biochemical structure, making it useful in conditions that require the dispersal or removal of inappropriate energetic imprints in the chakras.

Yellow rays carry positive energies to stimulate mental activity and the power of our mind. Yellow is used when there is a lack of physical or subtle-energy vitality.

Green, being midpoint in the colour spectrum, is neither a 'hot' nor a 'cold' colour. It brings balance, harmony and wholeness. However, do not use green if you are pregnant or have an issue with depression or cancer – in these instances, consult a qualified colour therapist.

Turquoise-blue has a strengthening and protective effect upon the physical body. It is an excellent colour ray to 'cool' any overactive chakras or to visualize as a means of protection around the whole body and auric field.

Blue is the colour ray that symbolizes inspiration, peace and devotion. It is used to slow down any body system or overactive chakra. Blue makes an excellent colour to visualize during meditation or to use in your healing sacred space.

Indigo is not generally used in colour healing, but it is the frequency with which the Third Eye Chakra resonates and takes one into deep levels of expansive, enhanced consciousness.

Violet rays enhance spirituality and self-respect. Its use with the Heart Chakra, or any chakras above it, uplifts the chakra in question and takes one into a realm of pure spiritual awareness.

Magenta is a colour really only seen as light – sometimes visible at sunset. The magenta ray used with the Heart Chakra, or any chakras above it, releases old ideas and conditioning in the chakra in question. It clears and uplifts it, dissolving rigidity and leading to personal spiritual evolution. Magenta is particularly appropriate to use with the higher chakras, such as the cosmic and transpersonal ones. You can read more about these chakras on page 219.

Developing my ESP abilities

Extra-sensory perception (ESP) originates at the Third Eye Chakra, assisted by the two minor chakras at the temples. Taking your time to work through all the exercises in this book, at least twice for each one, will gradually and naturally open your ESP abilities. Regular deep and complete relaxation (such as that taught in this workshop-in-a-book – see page 110), visualization and meditation are key to this process.

Different types of ESP

- The skill to see beyond the physical world is known as 'clairvoyance' – clear seeing.
- Hearing sounds or voices not in the physical world is 'clairaudience' – clear hearing.
- Sensing smells and perfumes not of this world is 'clairsentience' – clear feeling.

Some people appear to be born with these skills, and if these are recognized and allowed to develop, they may work as clairvoyants, mediums or healers. Others have the ability to see fairies or angels, but were told from an early age, 'Don't be silly – they are not really there.' Children frequently perceive auras around people, believing it is the natural way to see things – and, of course, it is – but unthinking adults may take them to have their eyes tested!

In the future, many babies will be born to enlightened parents who will recognize the importance of encouraging, rather than discouraging, ESP. This will create a resurgence of it, linking mysticism, science and spirituality. Just viewing the range of books now available on these subjects, compared to 25 years ago, shows the fundamental changes that are taking place in human consciousness.

A word of caution

Opening up your ESP can make you vulnerable to people who do not understand these energies. At many levels of your being, you will be reflecting an inner Light. Within your social group, ESP may not be a skill that you should talk about unless you are prepared to stand your ground, come out of your shell and reflect this inner

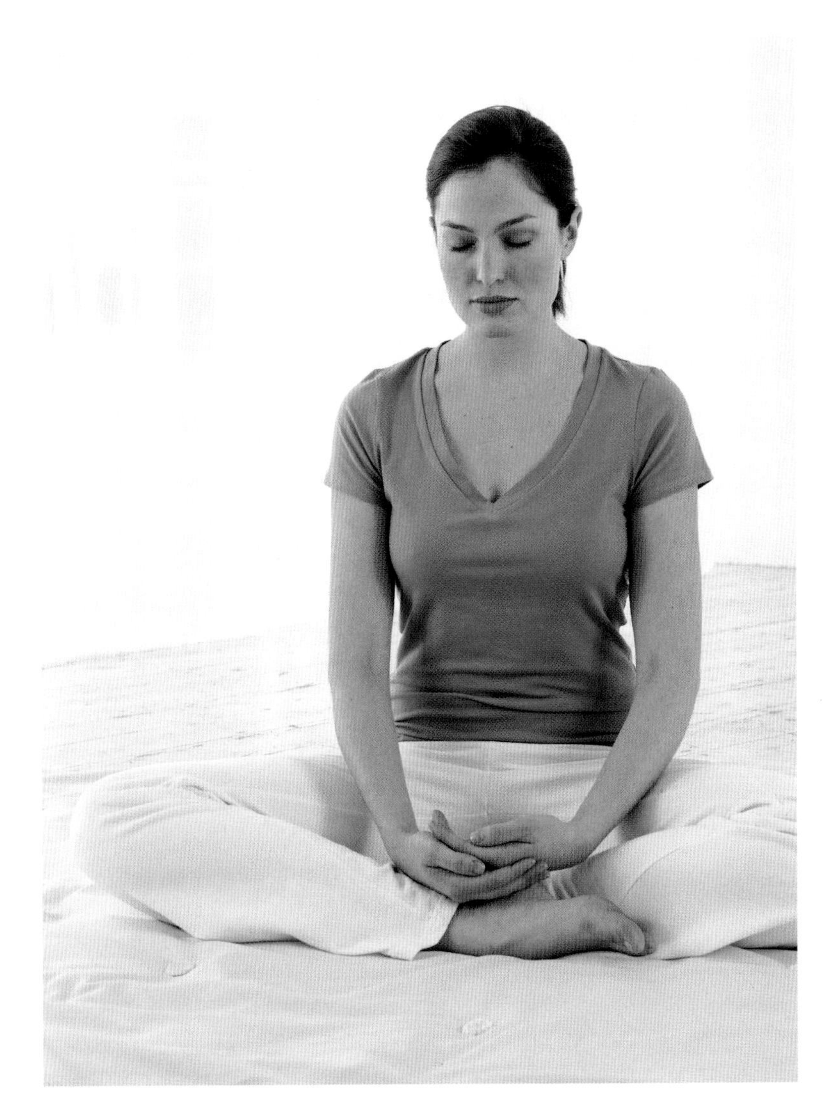

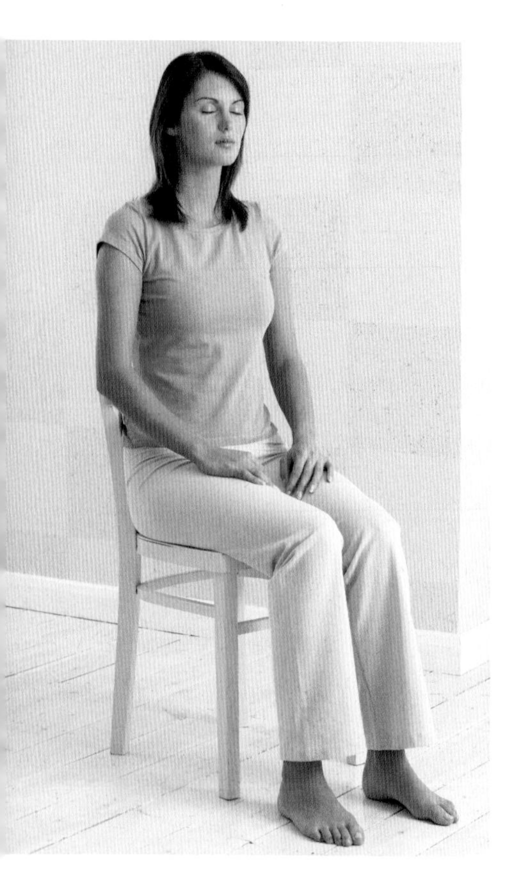

Light, which has gifted you with these abilities. When you really shine strongly as a beacon, it will attract all kinds of people and energies to you. Sometime these people actually prey upon your light energies, sucking into, drawing upon and trying to destroy your inner Light. While they may not be aware that they are doing this, you certainly need to be aware!

Protect yourself

Therefore consistently invoke a strong personal psychic protection. Visualize a cloak of deep-blue light that you can wrap securely around yourself. Or place a circle of clear white light around your body, 'drawing it' with a fingertip and then closing it up into a protective sphere/shell or egg shape of white radiance, which only positive energy can permeate.

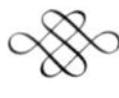

Work with your chakras now Turn to Exercise 27: Candle Meditation on page 197, for an exercise to develop your intuition and insight.

THIRD EYE CHAKRA EXERCISES

The following exercises develop the Third Eye Chakra or Ajna, which shows you other ways of perceiving the world, going beyond what you see with your physical eyes. They are intended to deepen your inner seeing, through visualization leading to meditation. They include a self-assessment that helps the release of negative patterns, a candle meditation and ways to protect your chakras.

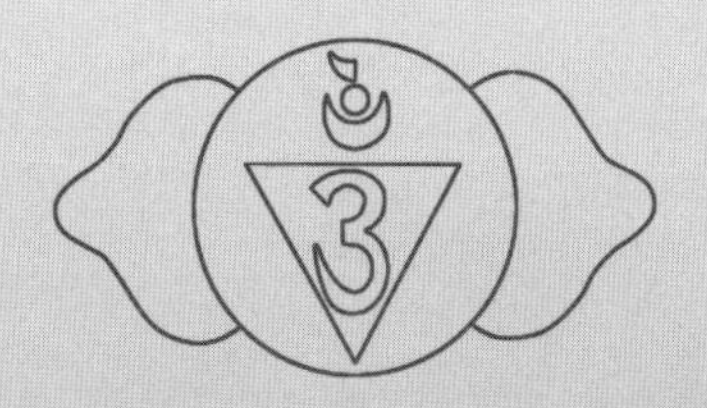

Developing intuition

Do this exercise before reading beyond this page. It will become a record of your Third Eye Chakra – showing your ability to engage with ESP – to which you can refer back in order to chart your progress.

Exercise 26 SENSING AND DRAWING MY THIRD EYE CHAKRA

You will need: a set of coloured pencils or pens (all colours, including magenta); keep the book open, ready to colour in the body outline opposite, which represents you (sign and date it before you begin).

- **To begin**, take five minutes sitting in a quiet place, breathing slowly, relaxing and closing your eyes. Now start to sense your body and your aura. Release any emotions that arise. Forget anything you have ever heard or read about chakras and auras. You are simply 'sensing' how your own unique energies are flowing at present. Check from your feet up to your head to pick up any little clues that your body is giving you. Sense your auric energy field around you as well. Now focus upon your Third Eye Chakra area, in the centre of your brow. What is it 'telling' you? What can you sense? Does it feel free, flowing, harmonious? Or is an old pain or trauma held there? Does it feel 'grounded' – or have you shut off all feelings and thoughts of this chakra?
- **When you feel ready**, open your eyes and – immediately and without thinking – quickly colour in the Third Eye Chakra area and any other parts of the body (and the surrounding page) as you wish. There is no right or wrong place to apply the colour: it is entirely up to you.
- **Read the interpretation** on page 196 after completing this exercise.

My sensing and drawing my third eye chakra experience

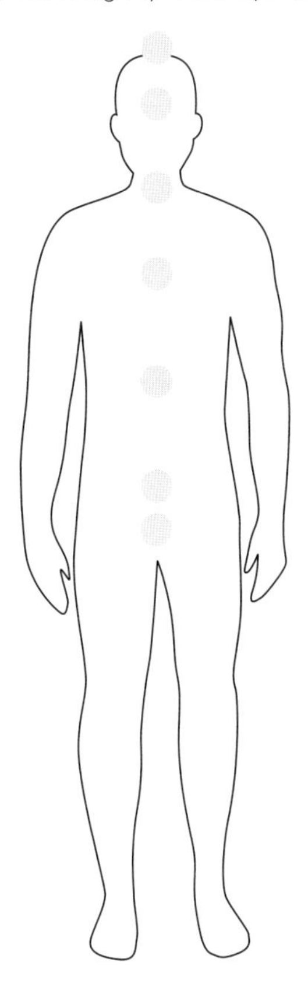

Date ______________________ Signature ______________________

Assessing my results for Exercise 26

A balanced Third Eye Chakra will show strong and vibrant colours in the blue to violet range. It will reflect your 'inner eye', your ability to engage with ESP, visions and deep transformative meditation. Balance shows your personal empowerment and respect for the life and spiritual paths of others. You will be outgoing, cheerful, relaxed, intuitive, demonstrating natural ESP such as telepathy or the ability to meditate easily. You may be a natural healer or spiritual teacher. You will be drawn to deepen your interest in metaphysical teachings.

An unbalanced Third Eye Chakra will show few or no colours, or possibly very strong and disjointed colours and patterns. These colours may be dark shades – black, brown or grey or a strong, dull red. When weakened, it will reflect depression, insecurity, dubious occult tendencies, fear of other situations or other dimensional realities. Overactivity of this chakra may make you egotistical, controlling, judgmental, sarcastic and a petty perfectionist.

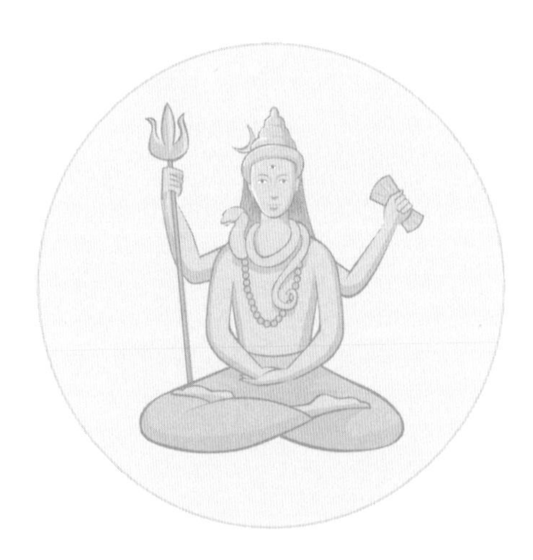

Developing insight

This is an ancient yogic technique called Tratakam, which helps to develop visualization techniques and brings great inner peace. You should do this exercise regularly to develop ESP and Third Eye Chakra sensitivity, but for no longer than 30 minutes at a time.

Exercise 27 CANDLE MEDITATION

You will need: a candle and a pen to record your results.

- **To begin**, sit in a dark room in front of a candle, placed about 1 m (3 ft) away from you at eye level. Ensure that you are sitting comfortably and upright.
- **Close your eyes** and take three deep, relaxing breaths.
- **Open your eyes** and look straight at the candle flame without blinking.
- **Close your eyes** when they become tired and, with your eyelids closed, look upward to your Third Eye Chakra.
- **There you will see** an inner image of the candle flame, and probably many colours. Hold this image for as long as you can.
- **Eventually** all images will disappear and then you can reopen your eyes. Be ready to record your experience on the next page.
- **Now consider** the questions on page 198.

My candle meditation experience

Date ______________________________

What did I experience when I closed my eyes? ______________________________

____

What does this teach me? ______________________________

____

Was this exercise easy/difficult (indicate which) ______________________________

____

Date ______________________________

What did I experience when I closed my eyes? ______________________________

____

What does this teach me? ______________________________

____

Was this exercise easy/difficult (indicate which) ______________________________

____

Overlaying a pattern of perfection

We all occasionally need some help to see clearly what is limiting us. Our physical and energy bodies – comprising the chakras and aura – accumulate all of life's experiences, both those that we consider good and those we consider bad. They may be held in rigid horizontal banding that prevents upward flow through the whole body field. Sometimes they linger as negative patterns that need to be identified and then released, through the methods explained in this book. In place of negative patterns we can choose to consciously overlay a pattern of perfection, comprising light-encoded frequencies for the well-being of our mind, body and spirit.

Exercise 28 RELEASING NEGATIVE PATTERNS

You will **need:** a pen to record your results.

- **To begin,** remain focused and silent for a moment.
- **Assess** the simple statements on pages 200–201. Be honest with yourself and circle the statement that reflects your answer.
- **Once you have considered** all the statements, count the number of nos you scored and read what that means.
- **Think** about how you can remedy any negative patterns and turn those answers into positive statements. Record those statements on the form on page 202.

My releasing negative patterns experience

Date ____

Take a while to assess the following simple statements. Be honest with yourself.

Circle the relevant answers below:

- I can relax easily Yes / No / Sometimes
- I feel comfortable in my body Yes / No / Sometimes
- I can use my mind creatively Yes / No / Sometimes
- I feel comfortable with spiritual concepts Yes / No / Sometimes
- I enjoy my own company Yes / No / Sometimes
- I enjoy the company of other people Yes / No / Sometimes
- I try not to judge other people by appearances Yes / No / Sometimes
- I have an open mind Yes / No / Sometimes
- I have a good and accurate memory Yes / No / Sometimes
- I can concentrate well Yes / No / Sometimes
- I look after my body Yes / No / Sometimes
- I appreciate my home/family/friends Yes / No / Sometimes
- I like to help other people Yes / No / Sometimes
- I have a positive self-image Yes / No / Sometimes
- I see the best in all situations Yes / No / Sometimes

- I have useful premonitions *Yes / No / Sometimes*
- I go to sleep easily *Yes / No / Sometimes*
- I have colourful and exciting dreams *Yes / No / Sometimes*
- I can visualize something easily *Yes / No / Sometimes*
- I enjoy being in Nature *Yes / No / Sometimes*
- I often meditate *Yes / No / Sometimes*

How many 'Nos' did you score? Record your score here ______________________

- If you answered 'No' to any of these statements, you are holding some unhelpful patterns in your energy body (chakras and aura).

- If you answered 'No' to five to ten of these statements, you need to work upon these aspects.

- If you answered 'No' to ten or more of these statements, you are holding some seriously unhelpful patterns in your energy body that will ultimately affect your physical body. It means that your personal vision is compromised and you would be wise to open yourself to the wonder of life – and make an extra effort to undertake the exercises in this workshop-in-a-book at least twice each, until you feel you have learned the lessons that you need at soul level.

- Think about how you can remedy the situation and record your thoughts on page 202.

Write here what you intend to do to remedy the situation, by making positive statements. (For example, 'I will be open to the ideas of other people and constructive in my responses'.)

Checking my Third Eye is balanced

This exercise uses a pendulum to check whether your Third Eye is balanced. As recommended on page 18, try to build up empathy and confidence in your pendulum, so that it can be used reliably to determine degrees of activity in each of your chakras. *Remember to avoid holding the pendulum over a chakra*, particularly if it is a crystal one – instead, point a finger of the other hand toward and near the chakra in question. This ensures that the pendulum doesn't falsify the reading.

Below are just some of the questions you may ask. Or how about asking if you need aromatherapy or sound healing exercises? Any questions that you ask must have only 'Yes' or 'No' answers.

Exercise 29 DOWSING THE THIRD EYE

You will need: a pendulum, and a pen to record your results

- **To begin**, remain focused and silent for a moment.
- **Then ask** the following questions:
  'Does this chakra require balancing?'
  'Is balance required on a physical level?'
  'Is balance required on a mental/emotional level?'
  'Is balance required on an energy level in my auric field?'

  It is also relevant to ask:
  'Is this chakra overactive or underactive?'
  'Is colour-breathing required?'
  'Is crystal balancing required?'
  'Is a change in my lifestyle required?'

- **Record your pendulum results** on the following page (date and sign them), so that you can begin to see repeating (or varying) patterns of chakra activity. You may dowse just the Third Eye Chakra, or you have space there to record the condition of all your chakras, if you wish. You can also compare the effects that various methods shown in this book have upon the chakras, by dowsing before and after any balancing work. It becomes very exciting when you do this, because you can start to see positive results.
- **As an optional method of dowsing**, use a blank 'body outline' (see pages 238–49). Sign it (this is your 'witness' or energy imprint). With the understanding that this body outline represents you, rest your index finger on each chakra in turn. Hold the pendulum in the other hand, well away from your physical body. Ask the questions given above. Record and date your results.

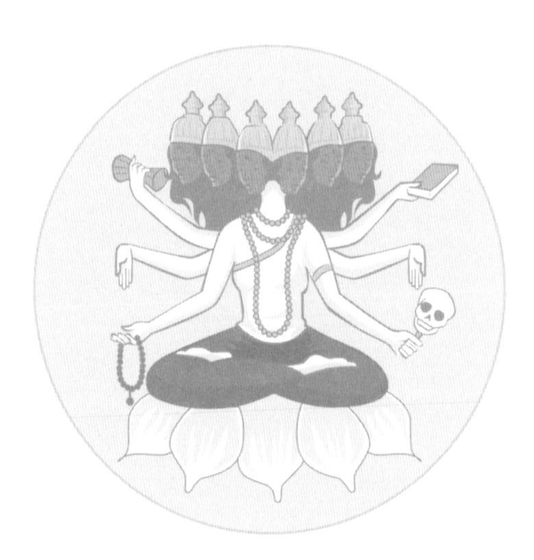

My dowsing the third eye experience

Date ______________________ Signature ______________________

- Does this __________ Chakra require balancing? Yes / No
- Is balance required on a physical level? Yes / No
- Is balance required on a mental/emotional level? Yes / No
- Is balance required on an energy level in my auric field? Yes / No
- Is this __________ Chakra overactive? Yes / No
- Is colour-breathing required? Yes / No
- Is crystal balancing required? Yes / No
- Is a change in my lifestyle required? Yes / No
- Is this __________ Chakra underactive? Yes / No
- Is colour-breathing required? Yes / No
- Is crystal balancing required? Yes / No
- Is a change in my lifestyle required? Yes / No
- Ask any other questions that you wish to pose.

Circle the relevant states below:

Base Chakra	Balanced	Underactive	Overactive
Sacral Chakra	Balanced	Underactive	Overactive
Solar Plexus Chakra	Balanced	Underactive	Overactive
Heart Chakra	Balanced	Underactive	Overactive
Throat Chakra	Balanced	Underactive	Overactive
Third Eye Chakra	Balanced	Underactive	Overactive
Crown Chakra	Balanced	Underactive	Overactive

Recharging my Third Eye

Using crystals with this exercise is optional, but if you use them they will increase the energetic frequencies for your Third Eye Chakra as you experience the colour-breathing. You need to be in a place where you will not be disturbed for approximately half an hour – indoors is okay, but it would be even better to be outside in Nature. Protecting the energy of your chakras is vital for well-being, especially as your spiritual journey unfolds. Here it is suggested you use turquoise light since it is the principal protective colour.

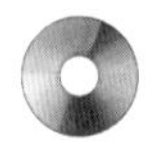

Exercise 30 COLOUR-BREATHING MY THIRD EYE CHAKRA

CD REFERENCE TRACK 2 (OPTIONAL) (TO FOLLOW THE SCRIPT, TURN TO PAGE 110)

You will need: one small clear quartz crystal with a point or five small, tumbled clear quartz crystals (optional), plus a meditation blanket to lie on.

- **To begin**, arrange the five tumbled quartz crystals (if you are using them) in a semicircle on the blanket around your head, or hold the quartz point (if you are using it) in the palm of your left hand, with the point directed up your arm.
- **Lie on your back** on your blanket and ensure that you are fully relaxed.
- **Close your eyes** and breathe slowly, visualizing your incoming breath as a clear, deep-blue light. Breathe deeply for a few minutes, focusing on your Third Eye Chakra. Experience the sensation of this coloured breath suffusing the area of your brow, head, eyes, ears, brain and Third Eye Chakra with energy.

- **Pause for a while**, then feel this coloured light spreading down your neck to your shoulders, relaxing them and bringing a feeling of total well-being. Again pause to let the deep-blue light-encoded frequencies permeate your physical body, energy body and consciousness.
- **Finally 'wrap' a cloak** of turquoise light around your whole body and auric field for protection.
- **Return to normal breathing** and, when you feel ready, slowly open your eyes.
- **Now consider** the questions on page 208.

Later, when you feel ready to do so, you may also work on the Third Eye Chakra with any of the other balancing methods mentioned on other pages of this book. Consult the chart on page 179 to ascertain which aromatherapy oil to use, which yoga postures, colour breathing, and so on.

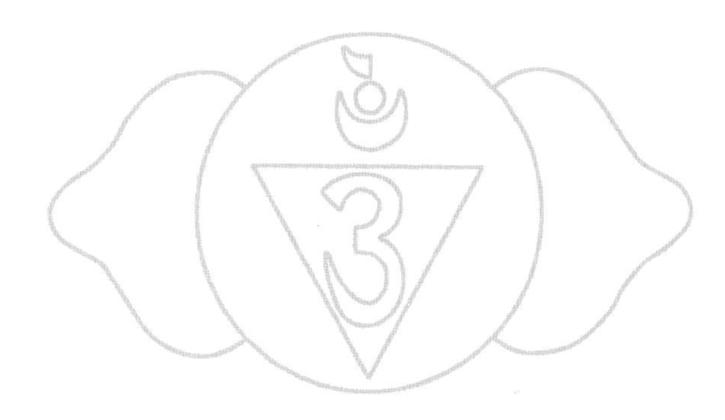

My colour-breathing my third eye chakra experience

Date ____

How well did I relax? Well / It was difficult / I couldn't relax at all

Does my Third Eye Chakra feel more balanced?
Yes / No / A bit, but then I lost the focus / Don't know

How did this exercise affect me? ______________________________

THE CROWN CHAKRA: SAHASRARA

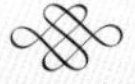 **Work with your chakras now** Before you read further, turn to Exercise 31: Sensing and Drawing my Crown Chakra on page 226.

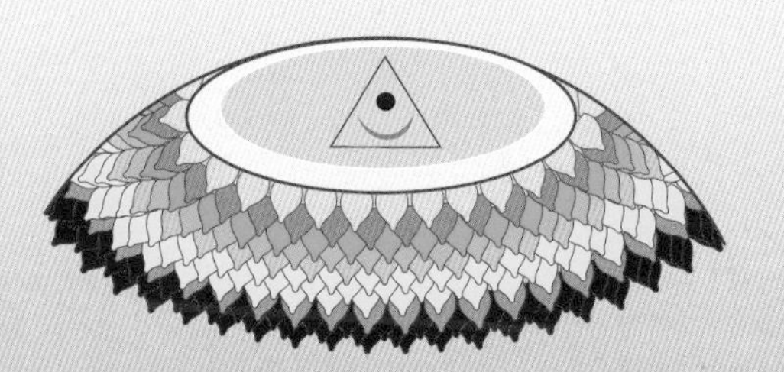

About my Crown Chakra

Keypoints: Resonates with Spirit and with pure white light flecked with gold and violet; has a connection to higher consciousness and inner wisdom.

The seventh chakra, the Crown, has Sanskrit name Sahasrara, 'the thousand-petalled lotus'. Here we finally reach a state of enlightenment when we choose to be released from the karmic 'wheel of life and rebirth'. In accordance with the traditional interpretation of karma, having recognized our divine self, there is no longer any reason to reincarnate.

It is written in the *Dhammapada*, a Buddhist collection of aphorisms or wise words:

'The traveller has reached the end of his journey. In the freedom of the infinite he is free from all sorrows, fetters that bound him are thrown away, and the burning fever of life is no more. He is calm like the earth that endures; he is steady like a column that is firm; he is pure like a lake that is clear; he is free from Samsara, the ever-returning life-in-death. In the light of his vision he has found his freedom; his thoughts are peace, his words are peace and his work is peace.'

The Crown Chakra activates and opens us up to higher consciousness, literally 'crowning' us with Great Spirit/Creator/Goddess/God. In yogic tradition, its many petals represent the spiritual work needed to perceive the source of manifest and unmanifest Spirit through the union of Shiva and Shakti at the Brahman Gate. In practice, this means that energies of duality, masculine and feminine, unite. Here lies the gate where the 'I' – the centre of our being – can transcend, creating superconsciousness beyond Time and Space. A process of unification occurs between human personality and a Higher Self containing tiny jewels of 'all that is, all that has been and all that ever will be', carried as soul seeds from one lifetime to another.

When we begin to glimpse what these yoga-inspired words mean, an enormous power is lit up in our minds. It may happen to you if you are serious about your spiritual practice. Once experienced, there is no going back – life is changed for ever, and everything is a play of subtle energies. In Tantric Buddhism, it is called the Rainbow of Liberated Energies.

CHART OF THE CROWN CHAKRA

Colour of influence	Intense violet/gold/white
Complementary light colour	Magenta
Colour to calm	Green
Physical location	Top of head
Physiological system	Central nervous system and brain
Endocrine system	Pineal
Key issues	Inner wisdom and ageing gracefully
Inner teaching	Releasing attachments to transcend Earth-bound karma
Energy action	Achieving Unity and Oneness
Balancing crystals	Amethyst and clear quartz
Balancing aromatherapy oils	Ylang-ylang, rosewood, linden
Balancing herbal teas	Chamomile or valerian (for sleep), a mix of wood betony, skullcap, chamomile, meadowsweet, hops and peppermint (for headaches), echinacea (for the lymph)
Balancing yoga position (*asana*)	Salamba sirhasana I (headstand) – advanced, Bakasana (crane) – beginners, Salamba sarvangasana I (shoulderstand)
Mantra/tone	OM in the note of B
Helpful musical instruments/music	Tibetan and crystal bowls
Planet/astrological sign/natural House	Jupiter/Neptune/Pisces/twelfth: challenges
Reiki hand position	Hold the back of the head
Power animal (Native American tradition)	Kachina Universal Spirit

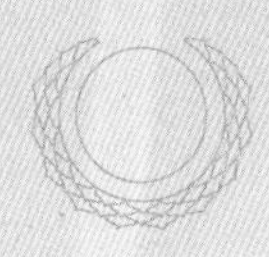

Body/Crown Chakra connections

The Crown Chakra is biologically linked to the whole endocrine system and to one of our most important rhythms of waking and sleeping. Unlike all the other six major chakras, this chakra opens upward like a funnel of energy and connects deep within the brain to the pineal gland, our biological clock. Among its functions are:

- Balancing the action between the pineal gland and the gonads (prostate/testes or ovaries/uterus at the Base Chakra), which work closely together to regulate sexual growth at puberty.
- Producing the hormone melatonin, which peaks during the 28-day menstrual cycle and is stimulated by light levels and particular wavelengths of light, although production of this hormone decreases in continuous light. It also regulates light photo-receptors in the retina of our eye and calms us down at night. During the hours of natural light, serotonin production in the pineal gland is at its peak, urging us into activity, so these two hormones work in a continuous circadian cycle.

More on melatonin

A modern disorder, SAD (seasonally affected disorder) is a type of depression reflecting unnatural cycles of sleep (natural rhythms take us to sleep at dusk and waken us at dawn). It is caused by melatonin/seratonin-cycle imbalance through the artificiality of street lighting, sleeping with the curtains closed or working at night. It can be improved by increasing the light levels in winter, preferably of sunlight, although a special daylight-simulation lamp can also be obtained.

As we begin to work with new awareness, cutting-edge medical research continues to throw more 'light' upon pineal-gland functions, validating chakra wisdom teachings – for example, the efficacy of meditating at night, or ideally at 3 a.m., when biologists confirm that melatonin production is at its peak and the Crown Chakra is active.

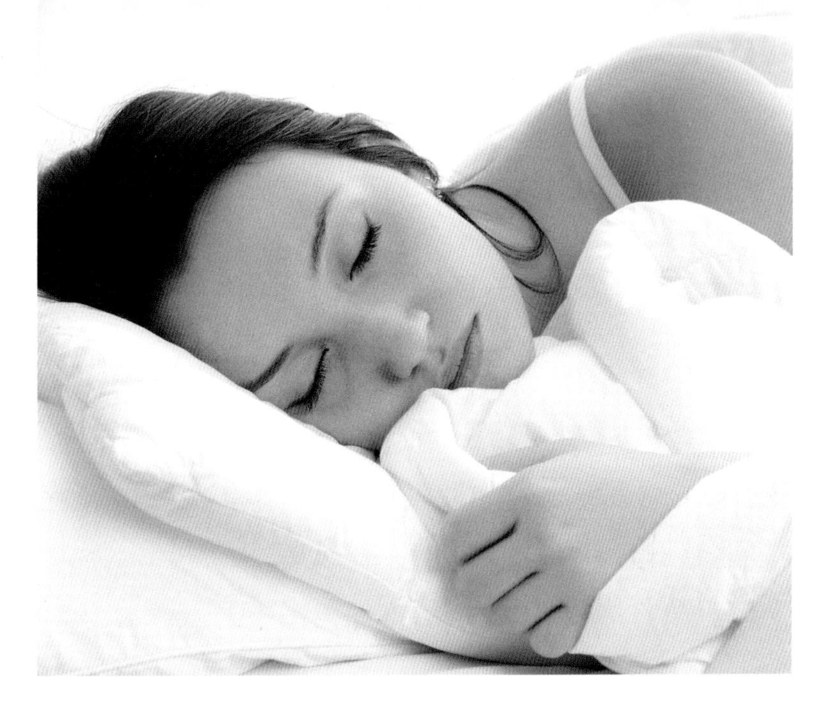

It is interesting to note that various hormones released by the pineal gland, including pinoline, are similar to LSD, producing natural hallucinations and heightened states of awareness. The pineal and adrenals also have a complex biological link that may influence stress levels, through the kidneys and abdominal organs, connected with the Solar Plexus and Sacral Chakras.

At both auric-field level and within our skulls, the Crown Chakra is linked to the pyramid shape of energy formed by the Brow Chakra and the Alta Major Chakra (see page 230 for more on this).

Did you know?

It is the pineal gland of some mammals that causes them to hibernate in winter in response to reduced daylight.

My Crown Chakra in balance

At the Crown, the 'Diamond Lotus', we ask, 'Am I committed to a daily spiritual practice?' If so, it is likely that the harmoniously balanced energies of all the chakras will flow upward to illuminate the Crown. In the past the aura of a saint was shown as a golden halo around the head, indicating development of their Crown Chakra.

The Crown is where we finally liberate consciousness that was previously attached to our physical body. We open up an ability to come into a state of 'superconsciousness' that is both personal and interpersonal, of this world and of other worlds, of this dimension and other dimensions. To achieve this we choose to release ego-driven self-created identity and liberate our wisdom inheritance. On an everyday level this means great challenges. If we let go of something, do we immediately replace it with something else? Or can we let go in order to find ourselves? Letting go of attachment requires us to see life simply as it is – not to embellish it with what is outside our control, but to be open to the many possibilities and energies that stream into our planet from all parts of the cosmos.

Using symbolic language

At the Crown, of necessity, we must turn to metaphysical, deeply esoteric language. Such specialized language was developed thousands of years ago in the Indian subcontinent by practitioners of yoga and related disciplines. It was written in the form of Sanskrit and is still used today for sacred texts that require complex spiritual concepts to be expressed. Using this symbolic language, we visualize our chakras as the lotus, whose roots are in the mud and whose flowers (similar to water lilies in appearance) reach skyward. Ask yourself these questions:

- Do I have a daily spiritual practice?
- Have I learned the lessons of the Base Chakra? Am I well rooted?
- Have I grown through the emotional 'mud' of the Sacral Chakra? Is the

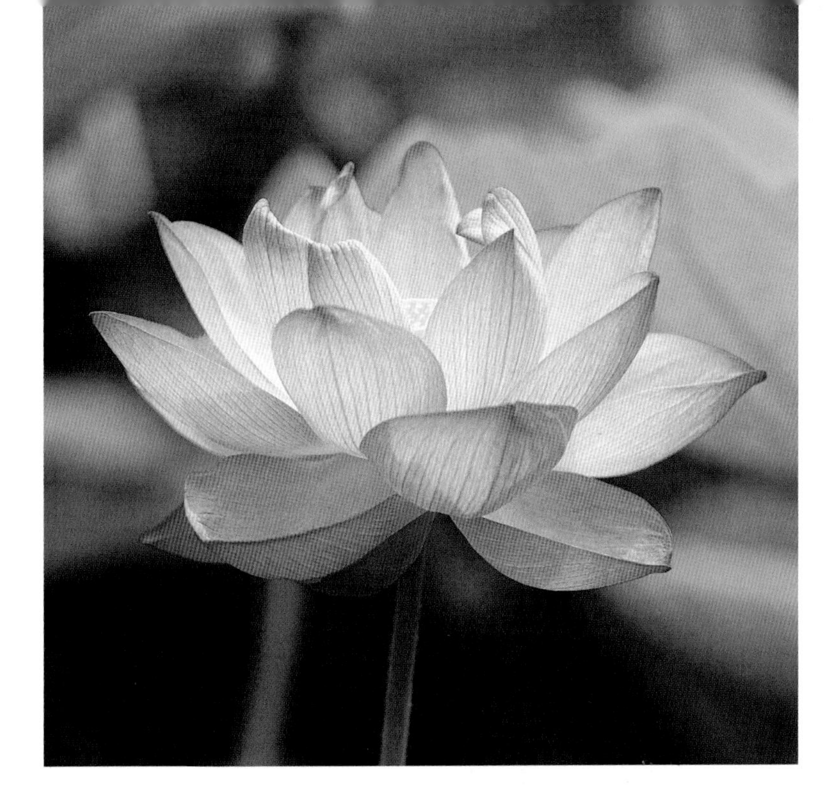

growing shoot of my life strong, straight and well intentioned as I reach for the next chakra?

- Have I allowed the physical and spiritual sun to shine upon my growth as I reached for the light at my Solar Plexus?
- Have I nurtured a precious flower bud with love in my Heart Chakra? Is that love given unconditionally to all beings?
- Can I authentically and honestly express myself through my Throat Chakra?
- When I visualize the lotus flower bud opening at my Third Eye, what does this look like?
- Can I stand fully receptive, vulnerable as an open flower, reflecting my inner and outer light at the Crown Chakra?
- Am I prepared to transcend ecstasy to reach Divine Bliss?

"Believe in miracles."

Ancestral imprints

Do you think you know your ancestors? How far back in your mother or father's line can you go: can you recall the full names of your grandmothers, great-grandmothers, great-great-grandmothers and grandfathers? Probably not. This probably reflects how, in our modern world, we give them very little significance. But many indigenous peoples can recall names stretching back for generations.

So who do we mean by 'ancestors'? Seven categories of ancestor are listed below. Their energetic imprints are embedded deeply in our auric field and seven chakras. It is up to us whether we are in harmony with this situation, or whether we wish to clear any negative imprints from our chakras.

Personal family bloodlines

The personal bloodlines of our mothers and fathers go right back to the start of time. We carry elements of these ancestors' DNA. We may well still have a living connection with some of them, or they had a strong guiding influence on our present lives. These may be held as inherited imprints of particular

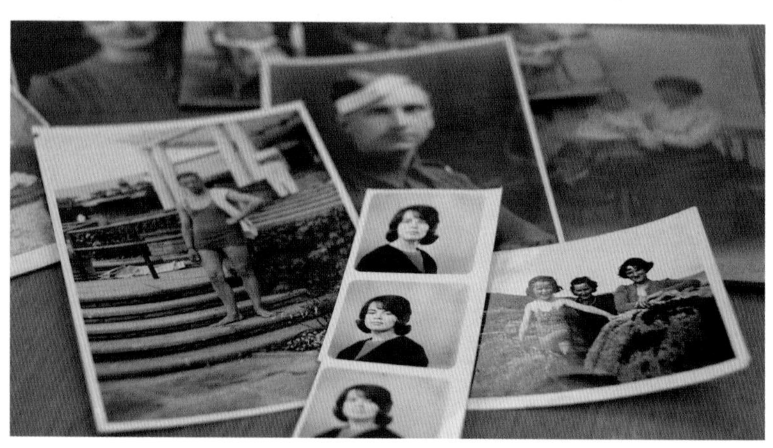

personality traits or dis-ease that we can eradicate at an energetic level. We associate them with red light at the Base Chakra.

National or tribal ancestors

Many of us are of mixed racial descent. Each of our ancestors made us who we are and brings with him or her the folk heroes and national leaders who have led their peoples over the ages. We may bless and release these ancestors, if we wish. We associate them with orange light at the Sacral Chakra.

Earth Spirit ancestors

These are essences of the land/s that have formed us: the elves, fairies, devas, sylphs, undines, salamanders, little people, the Tolilahqui (in Native American tradition) and so on. We may bless and release these ancestors, if we wish. We associate them with yellow/gold light at the Solar Plexus Chakra.

Mythic ancestors

These are supernatural beings in different world creation myths, which created Earth and the first human beings. These ancestors were usually born of both Earth and the stars. In Celtic tradition they are 'the Shining Ones'; but also consider: Athene/Apollo, Isis/Ra, Shakti/Shiva, Quetzalcoatl/Ixchel, plus aspects of the Great Mother Goddess – for example, Celtic: Brigit, Indian: Kali-ma, Egyptian: Hathor, Norse: Freya, Native American: Buffalo Calf Woman.

Our mythic ancestors may influence us strongly. Since some energies associated with them seem to us today to have been violent or war-like, you should only ever invoke the presence of those who will come to you in a peaceful, good way to guide your present life. We associate them with green light at the Heart Chakra.

Personal spirit ancestors

They are the beings that we once were in our karmic memories, our past lives. Included in this category are our parallel lives (past, present and future), the angelic influences that guided (and continue to guide) us, as well as spiritual masters or females to whose lineages we have been aligned. From a shamanic perspective, they are also spirit animals or clan spirits that guided our past lives. We may bless and release these ancestors, if we wish. We associate turquoise light with spirit ancestors at the Throat Chakra.

Star-people ancestors

These ancestors guided and mated with humans, seeded or in other ways influenced our DNA, our bodies and spiritual direction. They are star people with whom we feel a particular resonance – for example, those from the Pleiades or Sirius. Remember to ask for any extra-terrestrial ancestors to come 'in a good way, with good intent'. We associate them with blue light at the Third Eye Chakra.

Ascended-being ancestors

These are profound guiding influences, including Krishna, the Buddha, Mohammed and Jesus, as well as the Archangels. Their positive influences continue to guide many millions of people. Their aim? Unification with the Source! Our present life direction is subtly guided by them. We associate them with violet light, and within our luminous field the energetic imprints of beneficial ancestors merge into white light.

Clearing imprints

If you sense that you are in any way influenced by ancestral blockages, probably generated by deep trauma, then clear each chakra in turn, beginning with the Base Chakra. In your sacred space, light a candle and say out loud: 'I ask the ancestors to come to me in a good way.'

Focus upon flooding the chakra with the appropriate coloured light, as mentioned above. Say, 'I ask those ancestors who carry negative imprints in my energy field to leave me now.' Then seal each chakra in turn with an equal-armed cross of light and say, 'I ask the ancestors who come to me in a good way to remind me of the wisdom of the Ages that is within me, and to seal it within this chakra.'

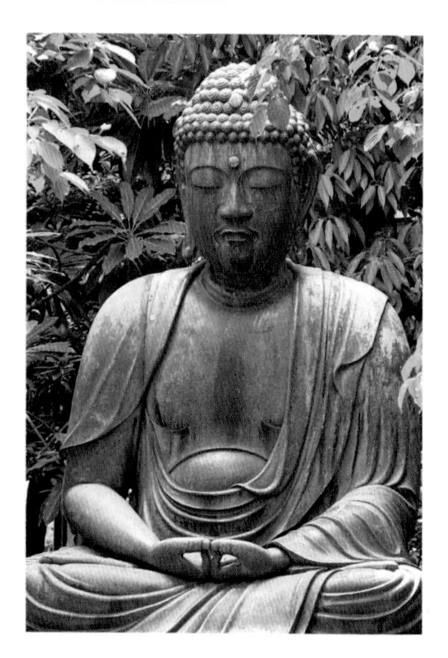

Reaching beyond the seven chakras

Applying a visionary perspective to the Indian chakra tradition, we can see how it has been a great and wise teaching for the past 2,000 years – but today humanity is rapidly evolving. Time appears to be speeding up. We are in the last few years of a great cycle of time spanning 26,000 years and a shorter 5,125-year period within it, which began during the Neolithic era and will end, according to the Maya wisdom teachers of Central America, in December 2012. They do not predict an apocalyptic end to our planet at that time, but rather a period of preparation, of clearing out the old, while humanity is confronted with difficult choices. A new cycle of time will then begin, when fresh patterns of life on Earth will be established. What they are depends upon the choices we make concerning the values by which we live.

Whether we listen to the Maya, Hopi and other indigenous peoples of the Americas, to the wise Hawaiian Kahuna, to elders and spiritual messengers from other aboriginal and tribal peoples or to visionary spiritual teachers within a Western context, we are hearing the same message. The cry is that everyone needs to wake up! We humans are being urged to take responsibility for ourselves and our beautiful planet. Our opportunity to evolve as a human race is *now*, and the outcome of this great 'experiment' in human consciousness depends upon you and me. There are two basic options – two spiralling timelines for us to pursue collectively at this critical time. Will we stay on the same timeline as our forebears and continue with our materialistic goals and destruction of Earth's resources? Or will we, with full awareness of the pulse of life that comes from the cosmos and regulates our chakras and subtle energies, choose to use the skills that we have learned in our lives to care for people and our planet?

At this decisive time in the development – indeed, evolution – of humanity, our spiritual skills take us beyond the Seven Chakra System and deeply into the significance of 12 chakras. One of these, the Earth Star, has only opened in very recent years, with the advent of environmental awareness. These additional chakras (particularly the Earth Star Chakra and three located above the head) link us to the whole planet, the galaxy and the cosmos. Developing awareness of them takes us on a positive timeline that ultimately stretches beyond Time itself, deep into an exploration of other quantum realities.

There is a natural limiting factor within these additional chakras – if you have not completed both practical and spiritual activations upon the traditional seven chakras, in accordance with your soul path, and are not living a good intentioned life from a heart-centred level, you are unlikely to find yourself open or receptive to these energetic gateways.

Conscious intention and meditation vertically align our supreme power as enlightened beings. Light enters

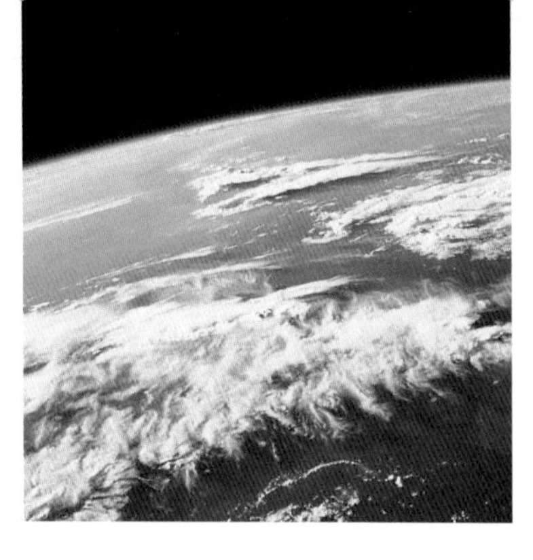

through the Stellar Gateway, Soul Star and Causal Chakra (see opposite) into the Crown Chakra. You may visualize it as sparkling golden light with a special quality of Divine Love, opening the heart to activate and ground energies at the Earth Star below. The response is for Earth energies to rise and meld at the Heart Chakra, sending out a strong vibrational signal, so that restructuring of our DNA and the journey to what we, as humans, have always intended to be can continue.

'Look with the opened inner eye. You will see everything you need, waiting to be shared.'

Optional advanced exercise Turn to Exercise 32: 'Be in the Flow' Meditation on page 228, for an advanced meditation.

Optional advanced exercise Or turn to Exercise 33: The Pyramid of Light on page 231, for another advanced meditation.

My 12 chakras

The five newly recognized chakras are transpersonal in nature. When awakened, we are taken beyond limited body/mind perceptions to interact with our wider environment and cosmic inheritance.

Earth Star Chakra

This was introduced on page 27. It is located just below our feet and is connected to the physical body by nerve endings, reflexology points and acupuncture meridians in the soles. It becomes activated when we allow our inner light to interact consciously with our environment and combine people care with planet care. This chakra is black and is not visible in the aura, unless we have strengthened and regained our intrinsic connection to the Earth, when it becomes a beautiful glowing magenta colour that 'walks' below our feet wherever we tread. Its purpose is the recreation of our bodies in preparation for restructuring DNA and, ultimately, luminous light-body ascension.

The Hara

This is closely linked to the Sacral Chakra, but in many people working with Eastern energy techniques it has

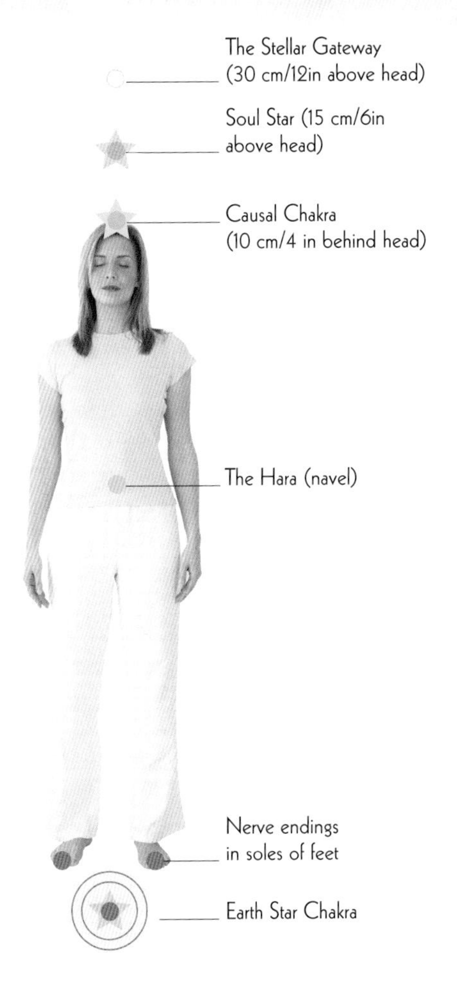

become dominant and is regarded as a separate chakra. It resonates with a strong orange-red colour of light. This chakra is balanced using tiger's eye or carnelian crystals.

Causal Chakra

This is located 10 cm (4 in) back from the Crown Chakra, lying just above the head and aligning with the spinal column. It helps development of the 'higher self' – an aspect of us beyond conscience. Conscience is conditioned, moulded and, at extremes, manipulated by the society in which we live. But the higher self knows, at core level, the right action to take in any circumstances because it is an expression of our soul. When we follow a path of unconditional love and repeatedly act selflessly, we are linked to our higher self in daily action.

The Causal Chakra guides our present lives, if we have released ego and opened up to Spirit – at which point it becomes a purifying filter through which we perceive life on Earth. It enables us to make good decisions and right choices for the benefit of the many, within an 'ocean' of inner peace and tranquillity. You will know when your Causal is balanced because your life will be a reflection of the peace that you feel in your physical and spiritual Heart Chakra. Crystals to enhance awareness of the Causal Chakra are celestite and moonstone, while kyanite directs positive energy and 'cuts' unwanted energy.

Soul Star

This is located 15–30 cm (6–12 in) above the head. Through energy impulses coming from the Crown Chakra, it transmits light-encoded information upward and outward to the Source. Reciprocally it filters incoming galactic information in order that it may be comprehended and acted upon at an awakened human level. It is believed that the Soul Star is where the soul rests immediately after death, before transition to other realities. Crystals to enhance awareness of the Soul Star are selenite, pink petalite or phenacite.

The Stellar Gateway

This is located a little above the Soul Star or is expanded an infinite distance into space. Full activation of this gateway will only occur when humanity is collectively ready to receive the inconceivably high vibrational energy of the cosmos. Crystals to enhance awareness of the Stellar Gateway are dark-green moldavite and Brandenburg crystal.

CHART OF THE 12 CHAKRAS

NAME OF CHAKRA	LIGHT COLOUR	PROPERTIES	LIFE LESSON
Earth Star	Black/magenta	Spiritual grounding point	Transmutation of fears
Base Chakra	Red	Physical grounding point	Establishing purpose on Earth
Sacral Chakra	Orange-red	Generative creative energy	Seeking balance with all life forms
Hara	Orange-yellow	Physical sustenance and strength	Balancing energy and Spirit
Solar Plexus Chakra	Yellow	Development of mental/ physical movement	Honouring wisdom in others
Heart Chakra	Green	Unconditional Love/ compassion	Honouring Divine Love
Throat Chakra	Turquoise blue	Verbal/artistic expression	Resonating with compassion
Third Eye Chakra	Deep intense blue	Inner sight, purification of thought	Completing karmic lessons
Crown Chakra	Purple/gold /white	Expansion of consciousness	Transcending physicality
Causal Chakra	Aqua	Conscious reprogramming	At-oneness with the solar system
Soul Star	Peach	Abode of soul after death	At-oneness with the galaxy
Stellar Gateway	Silver	Oneness, universal consciousness	At-oneness with the universe

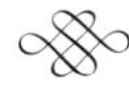

Work with your chakras now Turn to Exercise 34: Visualization for My 12 Chakras on page 233.

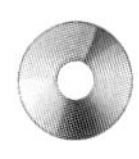

Work with the CD now Play CD reference Track 5 for the same visualization.

Death and transition

Death is a transition from one reality to another. Our lives in the energy field of Earth Mother. Finally a time comes when we have to release and seek independence in another dimensional experience and so some prefer to call death a transition – of energy, spirit, soul and consciousness. We're born through the Base Chakra and transit out through the Crown. At that point all bio-energy and body functions are released and we are declared 'dead'. Metaphysically the soul rests awhile in the Soul Star Chakra before moving on. This is why a tunnel and intense light are described by those who have had a near-death experience – they are seeing the light of the Crown and the three chakras aligned vertically above it, beckoning them into this other dimension.

A peaceful transition

Knowing this, we can assist in the transition of those we love, or in our own transition. At the appropriate time, consciously move energy up through the chakras and, finally, fully open the thousand-petalled lotus at the Crown. Infinite peace will result, which releases the soul into a great flow, like an enormous river, that carries it toward the Divine Light. A peaceful transition is greatly aided by playing soft music and talking to a loved one even if they appear to be unconscious. Sometimes we are at a loss to know how to use meaningful ceremony, so light candles and make the room comfortable for everyone present. Sometimes in our modern culture we are at a loss to know how to perform a meaningful ceremony that aids transition, particularly when the emotions are in full flow. If it is acceptable, place a quartz crystal pointing upward on the Third Eye Chakra of the dying person; position another just above their head, again pointing upward. This will encourage the upward movement of energy.

Use the ideas and teachings in this book with lightness and love in your Heart Chakra, expanding the wisdom acquired through insights at the Third Eye. Wisdom – different from knowledge – dawns through visionary consciousness. So look at life with an open inner eye. You will see everything you need, waiting to be shared.

CROWN CHAKRA EXERCISES

The following exercises develop the Crown Chakra or Sahasrara, taking you into the dimensions of Spirit whilst remaining on Earth. You may expand deep personal insights of an uplifting, transformative nature. plus the ability to meditate and identify with your life-path through numerous exercises. A guided Visualization for My 12 Chakras follows, complete with CD instructions, and drawing a record of your complete energy field.

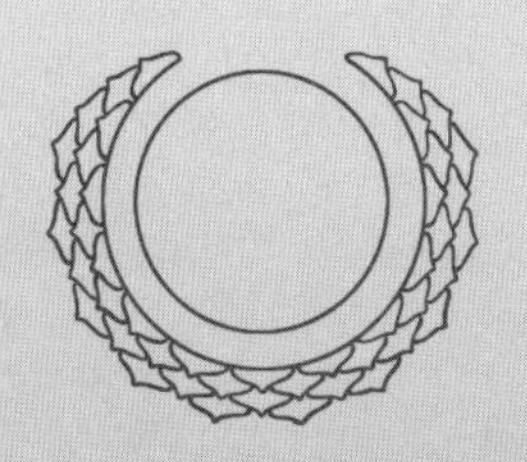

Developing intuition

Do this exercise before reading beyond this page. It will become a record of your Crown Chakra and your higher chakras, to which you can refer back in order to chart your progress. Your developing ESP may take you into deep perceptions.

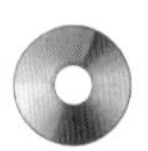

Exercise 31 SENSING AND DRAWING MY CROWN CHAKRA

You will need: a set of coloured pencils or pens (all colours, including magenta); keep the book open, ready to colour in the body outline opposite, which represents you (sign and date it before you begin).

- **To begin**, take five minutes sitting in a quiet place, breathing slowly, relaxing and closing your eyes. Now start to sense your body and your aura. Release any emotions that arise. Forget anything you have ever heard or read about chakras and auras. You are simply 'sensing' how your own unique energies are flowing at present. Check from your feet up to your head to pick up any little clues that your body is giving you. Sense your auric energy field around you as well. Now focus upon your Crown Chakra area, from the pelvis downward. What is it 'telling' you? What can you sense? Does it feel free, flowing, harmonious? Or is an old pain or trauma held there? Does it feel 'grounded' – or have you shut off all feelings and thoughts of this chakra?
- **When you feel ready**, open your eyes and – immediately and without thinking – quickly colour in the Crown Chakra area and any other parts of the body (and the surrounding page) as you wish. There is no right or wrong place to apply the colour: it is entirely up to you.
- **There is no need** to interpret the Crown and higher chakras. Their energy is so personal to you that you will probably require some considerable time to fully appreciate their subtleties.

My sensing and drawing my crown chakra experience

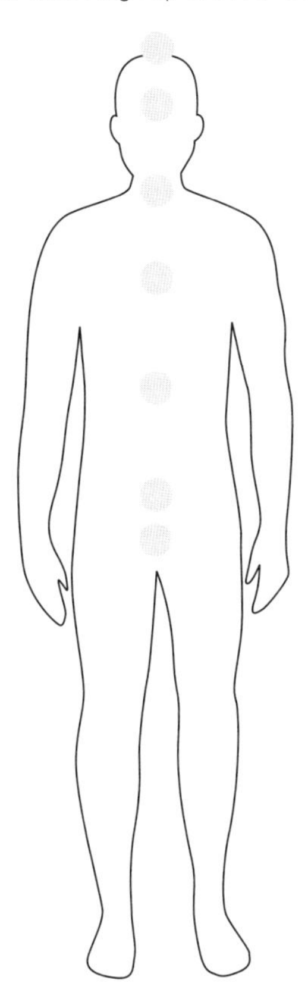

Date ______________________ Signature ______________________

Creating a bridge of energy

Our individual spiritual development brings a responsibility to contribute to the spiritual development of the planet. This meditation is termed light-bridging because it sends positive energies from your chakras to the four directions of the Earth in the form of cleansing light. It is best undertaken outdoors in a standing position. The purpose is to generate a bridge of energy between your Earth Star Chakra connection to the Earth and your Stellar Gateway to the cosmos. Only do this meditation for a short time, until you get used to it.

Exercise 32 'BE IN THE FLOW' MEDITATION

- **To begin**, face east. Stand outside with bare feet on the grass or earth. Activate all seven major chakras by visualizing your spine as a luminous column.
- **Send a strong 'root' down** from your feet through your Earth Star Chakra to the centre of the Earth.
- **Raise your arms** and ask to be filled with golden-white light. Imagine that your energy body has become so large that you can touch the stars. You are now 'in the flow' and bridging realities. Breathe deeply.
- **Lower your arms**, with the palms facing outward at shoulder level. Breathe golden-white light into your Heart Chakra, feeling it expand.
- **From your Heart Chakra**, visualize sending out light to the four compass directions of the Earth, turning around clockwise to do this. Start in the east; turn to the south, then west, then north. Imagine the light clearing all the places on Earth where there is pollution, despair or fear.
- **Feel joy** as you know that this work has been done, and gradually release the bridge of light.

My 'be in the flow' meditation experience

Date ______________________________

Place ______________________________

I felt ______________________________

____

____

Date ______________________________

Place ______________________________

I felt ______________________________

____

____

Date ______________________________

Place ______________________________

I felt ______________________________

____

____

Alta Major Chakra

The Alta Major is located at the back of the neck, on the base of the skull. It is one of our 'oldest' chakras because it holds distant memories and links to the rudimentary part of the brain. Yet it is of vital importance when we come to balancing a triad of chakras that comprise a sacred pyramid in the skull, because through the Alta Major we have inherited our ancestral survival patterns, our race memories and past lives. On the one hand, the energy here can be strong, heavy and dense, if our life-path has not enabled us to deal with these inherited traits. On the other hand, if we have cleared negative imprints here and filled the chakra with light, it takes its place in the pyramid, ready to transmute the alchemical gold at the centre. Try this advanced exercise to see the pyramid of light. Note that spiritual evolution – ultimately a spiritual rebirth – takes place through the Crown Chakra, while physical birth takes place through the Base.

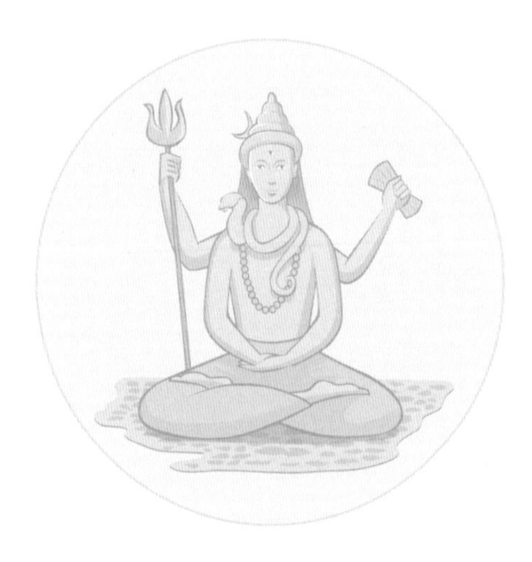

Exercise 33 THE PYRAMID OF LIGHT

- **To begin**, sit in a quiet place, feeling very relaxed.
- **Close your eyes** and begin to activate your head chakras by tapping your fingertips all over your skull for a few minutes in the following sequence: a line from Third Eye to Crown to Alta Major. Then in a circle horizontally from Third Eye to right temple, around the back of the skull to the left temple and return to the Third Eye.
- **Sit quietly** for a few minutes.
- **Concentrate on your Third Eye** and take a line of golden light from it right through your head to the Alta Major. Focus on the Alta Major.
- **Take a line of golden light** from your Alta Major right through your head to your Crown Chakra. Focus on the Crown Chakra.
- **Take a line of golden light** from your Crown Chakra right through your head to your Third Eye. Focus on the Third Eye.
- **Shift your focus** to the sacred golden pyramid now activated in your skull.
- **See the centre of the pyramid** being filled with sparkling golden light. It is the source of 'radiant ether' released through activation of the chakra system. Let this etheric light fill your head.
- **Release the golden light**, closing your Crown and Alta Major Chakras to an acceptable level of activity. Do the same in turn with the Third Eye, Throat, Heart, Solar Plexus, Sacral and Base Chakras.
- **Open your eyes** and be gentle with yourself for the rest of the day.

My pyramid of light experience

Date ______________________________

Fingertip-tapping helped awaken my head chakras. Yes / No

I was relaxed. Yes / No

I experienced ______________________________

____

____

____

____

Date ______________________________

Fingertip-tapping helped awaken my head chakras. Yes / No

I was relaxed. Yes / No

I experienced ______________________________

____

____

____

____

Guided visualization

Blue is the colour that brings peace. In the following visualization it is combined with golden light to balance your 12 chakras with your auric field.

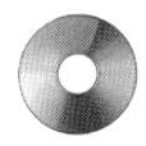

Exercise 34 VISUALIZATION FOR MY 12 CHAKRAS

CD REFERENCE TRACK 2 (OPTIONAL) (TO FOLLOW THE SCRIPT, SEE PAGE 110)

CD REFERENCE TRACK 4 (TO FOLLOW THE SCRIPT, SEE BELOW)

- **To begin**, lie down, preferably outdoors, but otherwise find a comfortable place indoors.
- **Imagine you are climbing** up the stone steps of a tall pyramid. You observe that it has 12 levels and a flat top with a small temple upon it. You reach the top and enter the temple.
- **Recline within the temple**, where an open circular window enables you to look directly up into the sky. See the vastness of the cloudless sky.
- **Wonder at the magnitude** of this atmosphere, which surrounds our Earth and stretches out beyond. Consider whether space is infinite or has a beginning and an end.
- **Consider how little** we really know about the galaxies and life beyond our own, and how small we are in this huge cosmic field.
- **Now concentrate on the sun**, taking a moment to appreciate its importance in sustaining life. Without it, all would be barren, lifeless and dark. Visualize a shaft of golden light pouring from the sun into the deep mysterious blueness of space. Let yourself travel within this golden light out into the universe. While you are doing so, a dark-blue light protects and holds you in its peaceful cloak.

- **In the immensity of space** you are just floating and moving gently. Without gravity you can effortlessly turn and look at the stars and planets. Each has its own colour of light and its own sound that blends with the whole, to create a 'symphony of the spheres'.
- **Let the colours and sounds** permeate your energy body, surging through your 12 chakras. They cause your physical body – each organ, muscle and bone – to resonate with its own perfect frequency of sound, creating wholeness within you.
- **Remember** that you came from the stars – and to the stars you will return.
- **Focus again** upon the dark blueness of space and consider your own spiritual path: is there a message for you?
- **When you feel ready,** travel within the shaft of golden light through the sun, then back to Earth. Become aware of your body lying within the temple. Descend the 12 levels carefully, step by step, and become once again fully present in your physical body, noting any changes to your chakras.

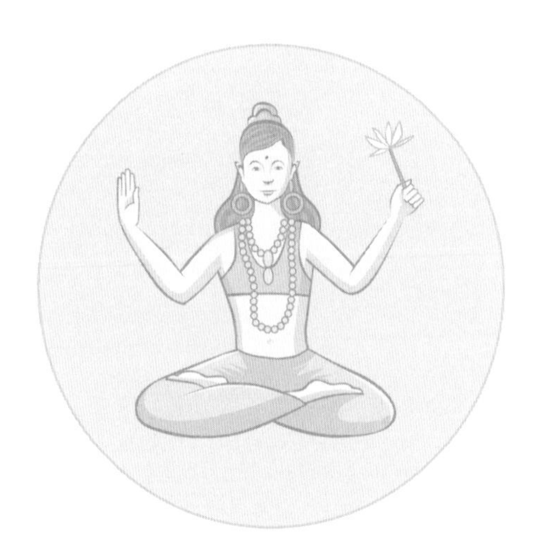

My visualization for my 12 chakras experience

Date ______________________________

I relaxed   Well / not very well

I could visualize the temple easily   Yes / No

I could visualize travelling in the shaft of golden light   Yes / No

Check out each chakra and make appropriate notes ______________________________

I also experienced ______________________________

Developing intuition

This final exercise will become a record of your complete subtle-energy system, chakras and aura, to which you can refer back in order to see the extent to which you have progressed. You may compare it with the very first body outline that you intuitively coloured in on page 35.

Exercise 35 COLOURING MY SUBTLE-ENERGY SYSTEM

You will need: a set of coloured pencils or pens (all colours, including magenta); keep the book open, ready to colour in the body outline opposite, which represents you (sign and date it before you begin).

- **To begin,** take five minutes sitting in a quiet place, breathing slowly, relaxing and closing your eyes. Now start to sense your body and your aura. Release any emotions that arise. Forget anything you have ever heard or read about chakras and auras. You are simply 'sensing' how your own unique energies are flowing at present. Check from your feet up to your head to pick up any little clues that your body is giving you. Sense your auric energy field around you as well. What is it 'telling' you? Does your auric field feel fluid and open – or have you shut off all feelings and thoughts of it? Check through your chakras one by one. How are they feeling?
- **When you feel ready,** open your eyes and – immediately and without thinking – quickly colour in your complete chakra system of the seven main chakras, plus any of the higher head chakras and minor chakras or parts of the body (and the surrounding page) as you wish. There is no right or wrong place to apply the colour: it is entirely up to you.
- **There is no need** to interpret this drawing of your chakras and auric field. It represents a snapshot of where your energies are flowing at the present time. Just write any comments below the picture on the next page, date and sign it.

My colouring in my subtle-energy system experience

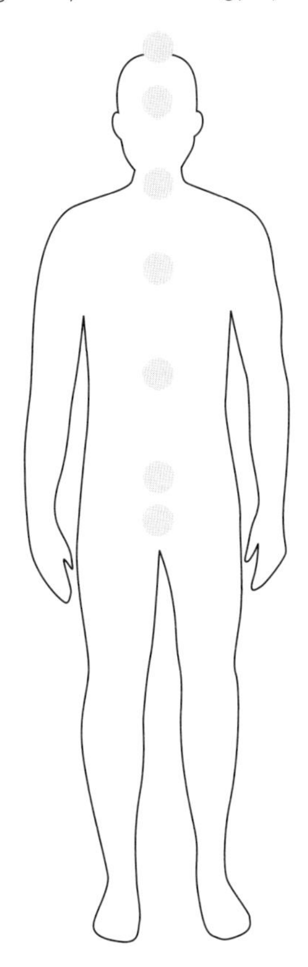

Date ______________________ Signature ______________________

BODY OUTLINE CHARTS

Use the following body outline charts to record your impressions when you sense the condition and balance of your chakras.

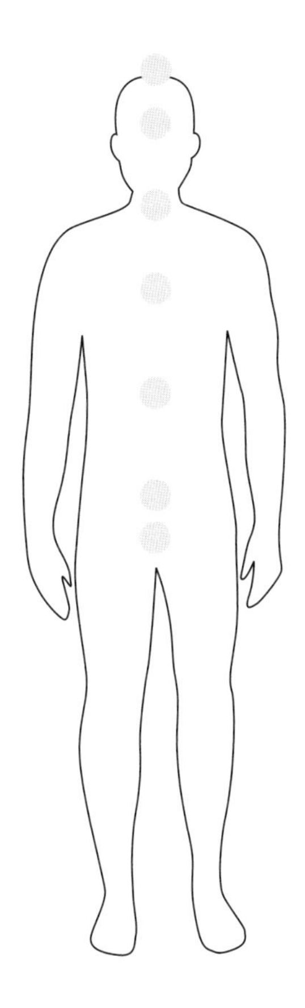

Date ______________________ Signature ______________________

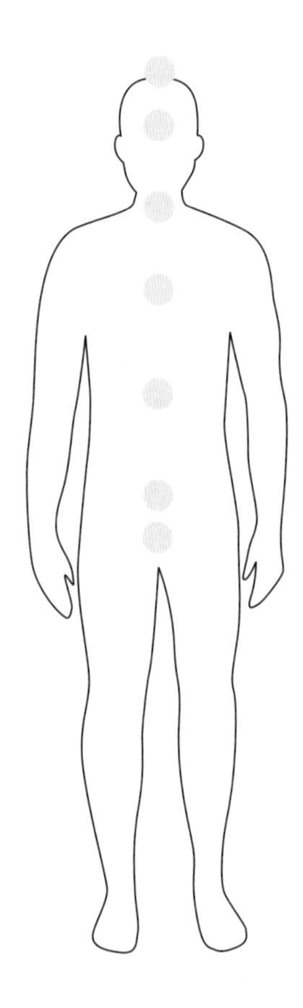

Date ______________________ Signature ______________________

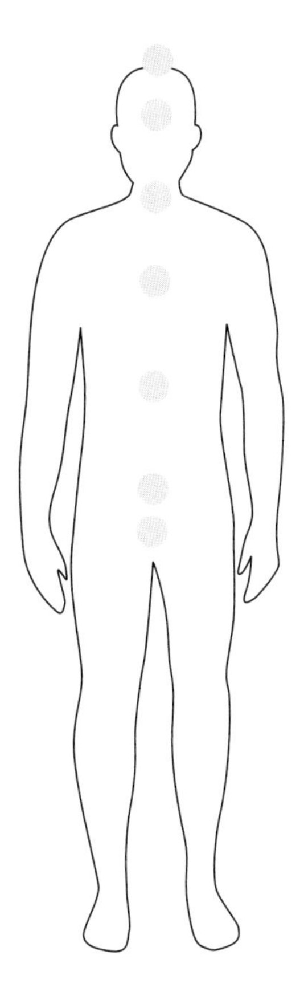

Date ______________________ Signature ______________________

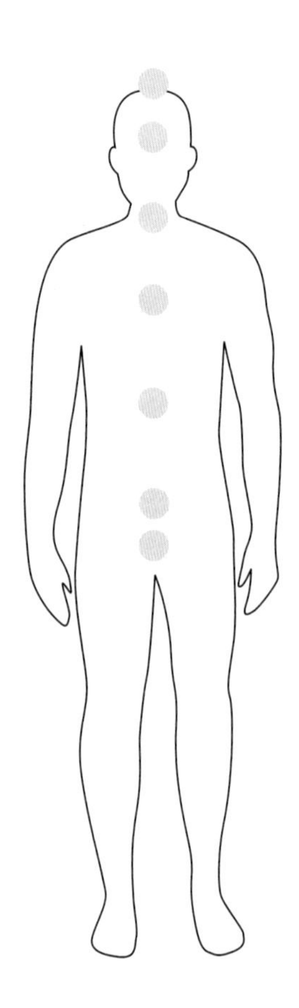

Date ______________________ Signature ______________________

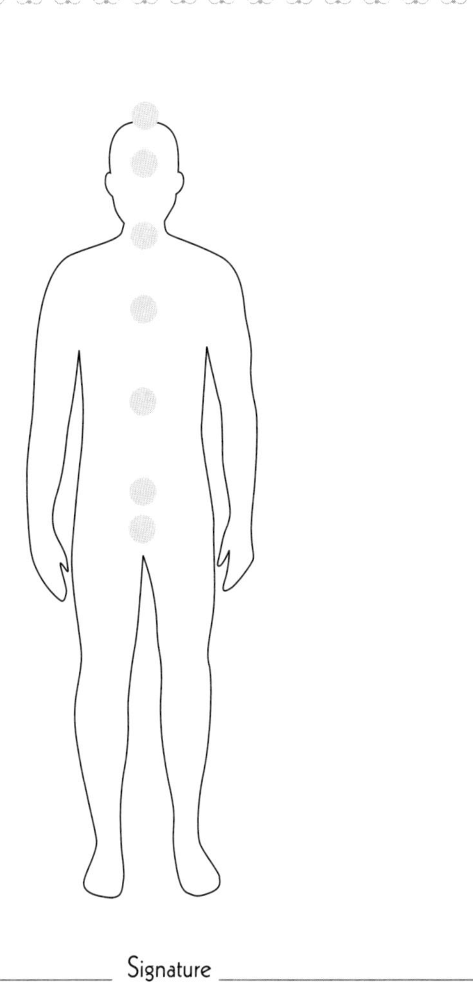

Date ______________________ Signature ______________________

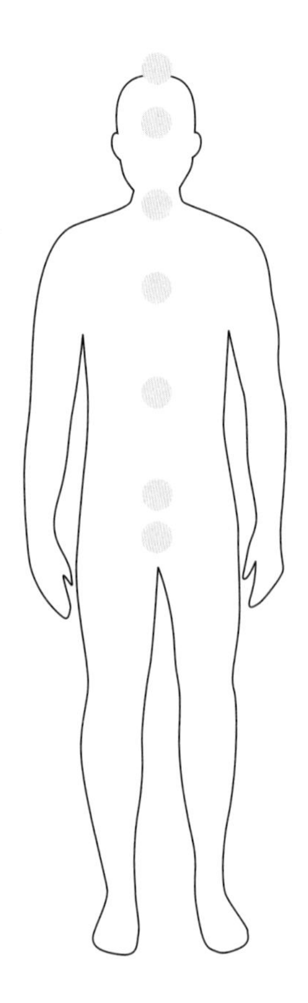

Date ______________________________ Signature ______________________________

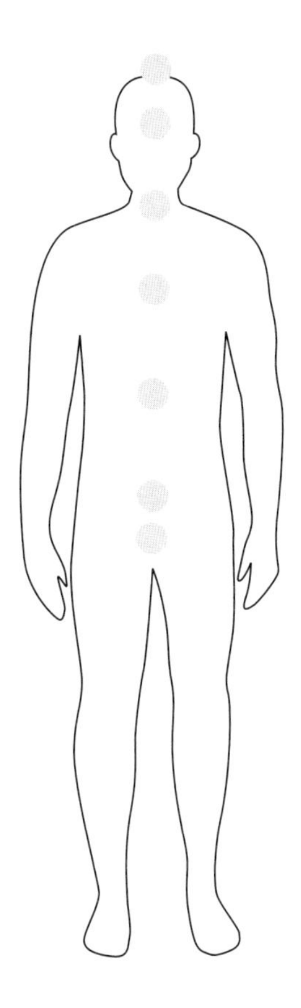

Date ______________________ Signature ______________________

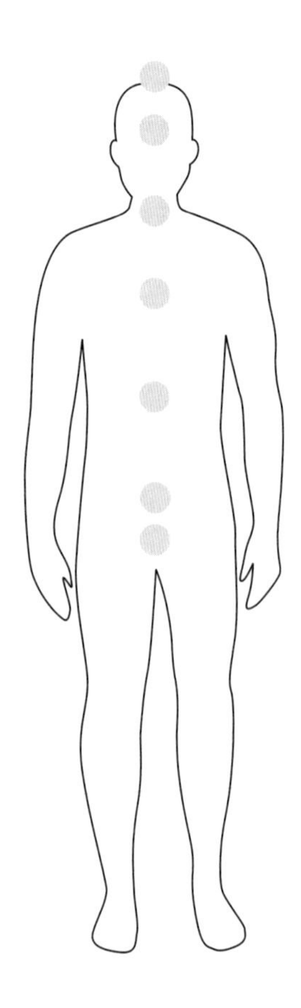

Date ______________________ Signature ______________________

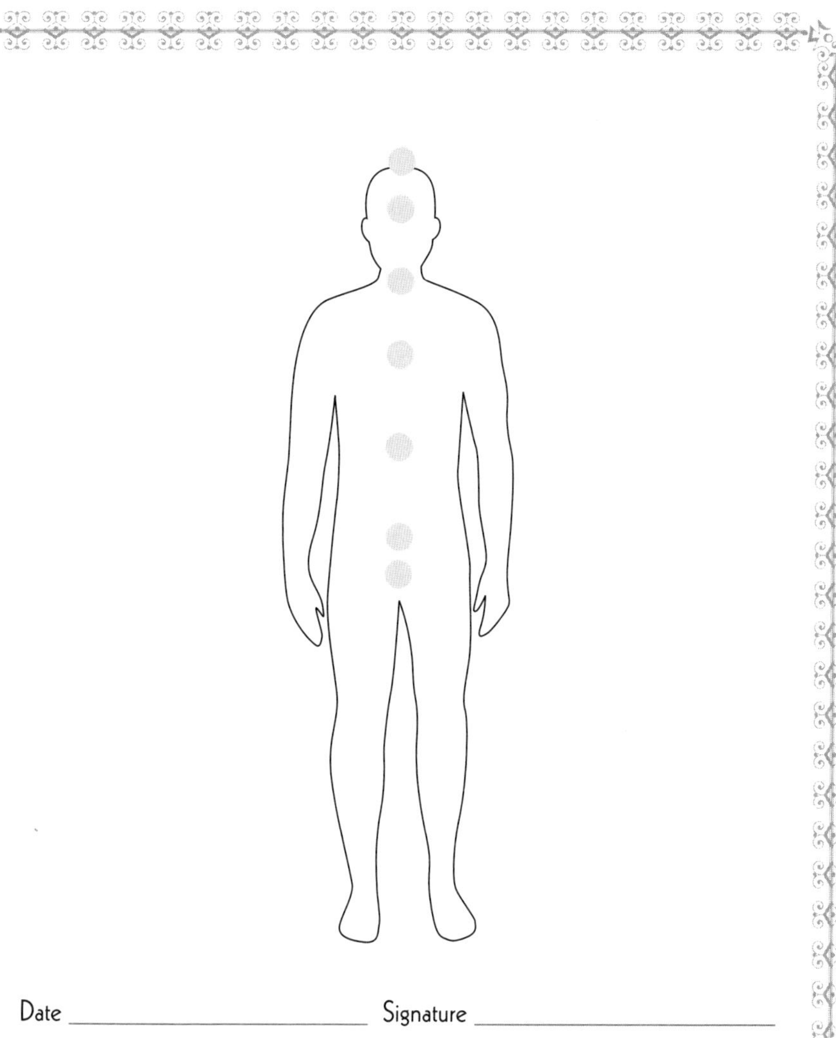
Date
Signature

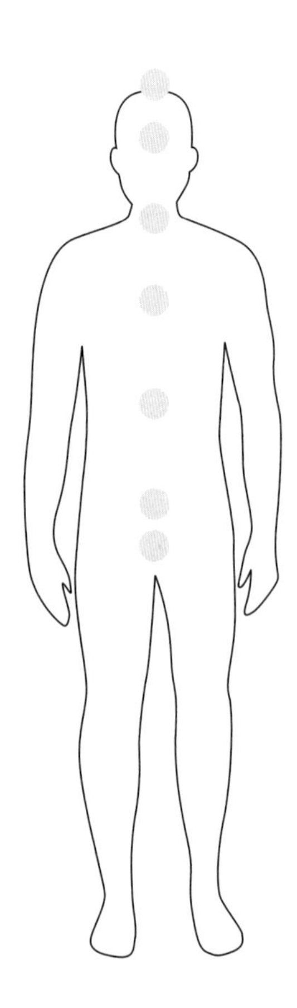

Date ____________________ Signature ____________________

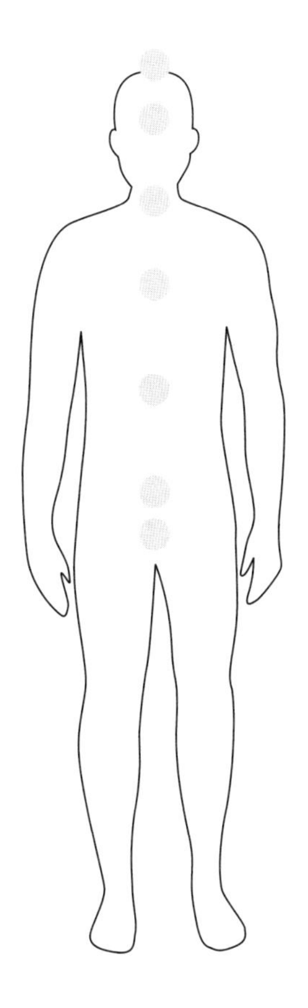

Date ______________________________ Signature ______________________________

Glossary of terms

Ancestral light body An aspect of our multidimensional self connected to our auric field.

Aura/auric field A subtle bio-energetic field of light surrounding a physical body, which, although not easily seen, may be sensed.

Being of Light An incarnate or disincarnate being or person, vibrating at high frequencies of light.

Body language Movements or expressions indicating our state of wellness and ease or disharmony and dis-ease.

Chi/ki A generalized type of subtle energy, identical to *prana*; a Chinese and Japanese term.

Clairvoyance Clearly seeing non-physical realms; closely associated with intuition.

Dis-ease Not being at ease in our body, and our body demonstrating that we need to rebalance it.

Ego A psychological term meaning one of the three main divisions of the mind; written here with a small 'e' to reduce its power.

Emotional imprint A subtle-energy pattern in the auric field and chakras.

Energy Medicine A wide-ranging and diverse holistic type of healthcare and healing, which provides treatment by balancing the human energy system; sometimes called Vibrational Healing.

Field of Life Part of the Quantum Field relevant to Earth life.

Force of Grace Force is an active energy, Grace is a special spiritual endowment or influence; in Hinduism, Grace is 'kripa', the ultimate key required for spiritual self-realization; in Buddhism, a state of Grace is attained through advancement on the Eightfold Path.

Healing crisis A rapid release of underlying causes of dis-ease that temporarily worsens a condition.

Inner child The vulnerable or playful part of our inner life/mind.

Karma Traditional: 'The wheel of cause and effect'; modern: an outdated attachment to Time, embedded deep in the fabric of our ancestral light body, causing compliance with archaic control mechanisms.

Kundalini Primal life energy, normally dormant at the base of the spine and having its roots at the Base Chakra.

Light Divine Spiritual Light, as compared to light (with a small 'l').

Luminous body/light body An 'awakened' and active human auric field.

Nadi A subtle-energy channel through which *prana* flows – similar, but not identical, to acupuncture meridians.

Prana A yogic term for a number of different types of subtle energy; sometimes called 'life-force'.

Quantum Field Interconnecting and interpenetrating energy fields of cosmic complexity and proportions.

Reiki A living path of spiritual healing rediscovered by Dr Mikao Usui.

Resonance When a particular body or system oscillates in its natural frequency as a result of impulses received from some other system that is vibrating with the same frequency.

Sanskrit A classical Indo-European language in which scientific, philosophical and religious ideas were expressed.

Subtle body An alternative expression for a person's auric and chakra energies; also the auric field, or a part or layer of it, such as the Lower Mental Body.

Superconsciousness Elevated human consciousness, both individually and collectively.

Yogi/yogic A dedicated practitioner of yoga/ pertaining to the practice of yoga.

Index

I

K

L

M

N

O

P

Acknowledgements

I would like to thank all the participants in my courses and workshops who, over the years, have helped me to develop and test the exercises in this book. Thanks, as always, to my husband and sound therapist Mikhail, who advised, researched and supported my writing.

Picture Acknowledgements

Alamy/Michael DeFreitas Asia 152; /Tetra Images 150. **Corbis**/Ocean 85, 125, 187. **Fotolia**/Coqrouge 29; /diez-artwork 1; /dngood 189; /Liv Friis-larsen 122; /Gorilla 55; /Barbara House 21; /Kathrin39 27; /kohashi 6, 215; /Mahesh Patil 91; /Richard Robinson 185; /Valua Vitaly 213; /WavebreakMediaMicro 88; /Zilotis 180. **Getty Images**/Martin Barraud 119; /B. Blue 127; /bravobravo 53; /Pascal Broze 116; /George Doyle 149; /Marcy Maloy 7; /Tom Merton 32; /moodboard 183; /Dejan Patic 157; /Trinette Reed 61. **Octopus Publishing Group** 63; /Colin Bowling 95 left; /Frazer Cunningham 13, 192, 221; /Janeanne Gilchrist 186; /Russell Sadur 17, 19, 57, 62, 93, 123, 191, 216; /Ruth Jenkinson 11, 21, 59, 159.

Commissioning Editor: Liz Dean
Managing Editor: Clare Churly
Deputy Art Director: Yasia Williams
Designer: Cobalt ID
Picture Library Manager: Jennifer Veall
Production Manager: Peter Hunt

CONTENTS

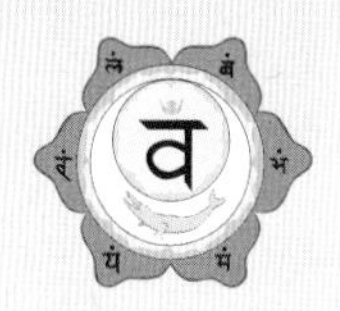

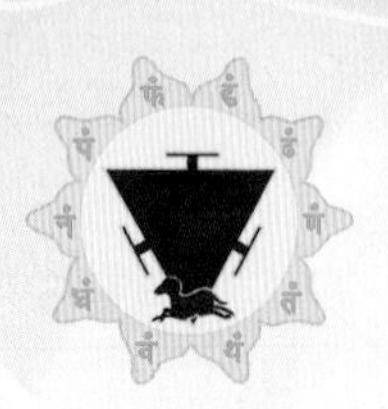

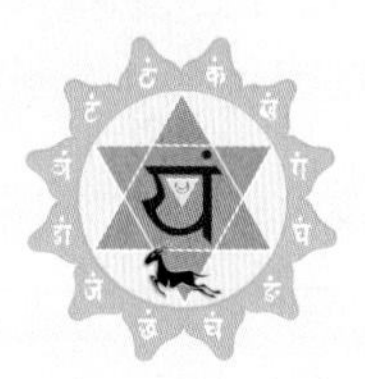

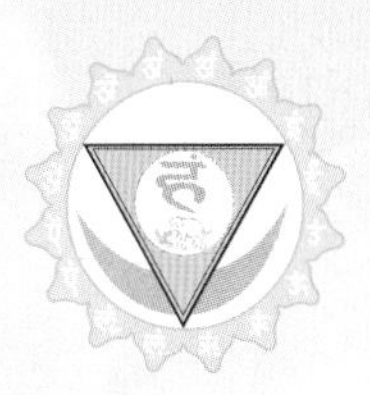

The Third Eye Chakra: Ajna 177

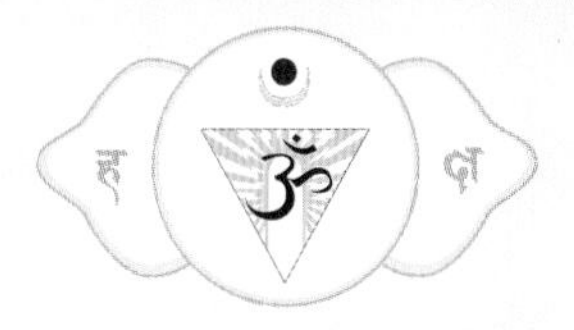

The Crown Chakra: Sahasrara 209

CD tracks

Introduction

Have you ever wondered about chakras, what they could mean for you and how you could understand them? By undertaking this workshop-in-a-book, now you can!

Perhaps you have heard chakras described in a yoga class as something rather mysterious, or have already started to 'tune in' to your own 'subtle body' (unseen, but discernible) energies. In my other books I gave a definitive guide to working with chakras. This book is like coming to one of my chakra workshop courses, because you will benefit from using the tried-and-tested exercises and visualizations, in combination with the CD.

What exactly are chakras?

Around our physical body there is an auric energy field (see page 10). Interacting with our body are spiralling energetic forces known as chakras (both their common and traditional Indian names are given in this book). Teachings originating in yoga refer to seven major chakras or body-power centres as follows, starting from the base of the spine:

1 **Base (Root) Chakra/Muladhara** – colour of influence: red
2 **Sacral Chakra/Svadisthana** – colour of influence: orange
3 **Solar Plexus Chakra/Manipura** – colour of influence: yellow
4 **Heart Chakra/Anahata** – colour of influence: green (or rose-pink)
5 **Throat Chakra/Vishuddha** – colour of influence: turquoise-blue (or sky-blue)
6 **Third Eye (Brow) Chakra/Ajna** – colour of influence: deep blue
7 **Crown Chakra/Sahasrara** – colour of influence: white, violet or gold.

From this sequence you can see how the chakras progress in the light spectrum. Each colour vibrates to its own frequency. We have seven major chakras and 22 interconnected minor and transpersonal chakras that connect us to the wider cosmic field – sometimes called the Quantum Field.

How to use the book and CD

After an explanatory opening section, as you come to each chapter in this book you will learn ways to clear, activate or balance the seven chakras, to facilitate body/mind/spirit harmony and wellness. You will be shown how to use a pendulum and crystals, do colour-breathing and visualizations/meditation and use aromatherapy and sound. Turn to the second part of each chapter for your personal workshop exercises, journal pages and recommendations on when to use the CD.

The CD provides musical tracks to accompany guided instruction for five of the exercises, which you will also find written as scripts in the book. Simply follow the instructions that you hear or, if you prefer, you can record your own.

Journal space is provided in each chapter to record your observations and experiences after the exercises. Remember to write the date. Try using keywords to get your thoughts down quickly. Keep some spare sheets of paper close by, if you prefer to make drawings of your experiences. When you are journaling, record your body's feelings, your thoughts and emotions, how relaxed you feel, whether your energy feels weaker or stronger, whether your sleep patterns are any different, whether your state of wellness is improved and any other information that you wish.

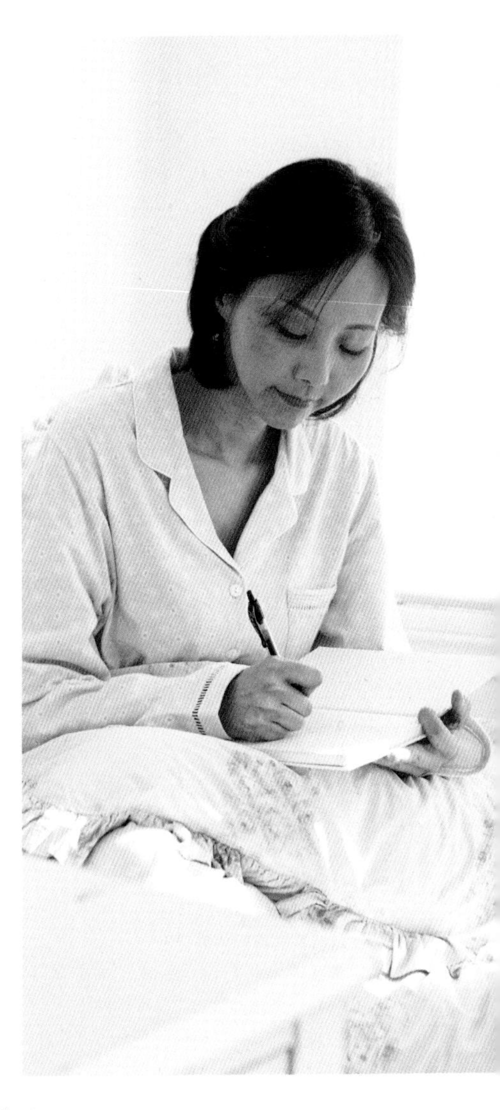

Symbols and recording your insights

Throughout this book you will find symbols to guide you in the next stage of your chakra exploration.

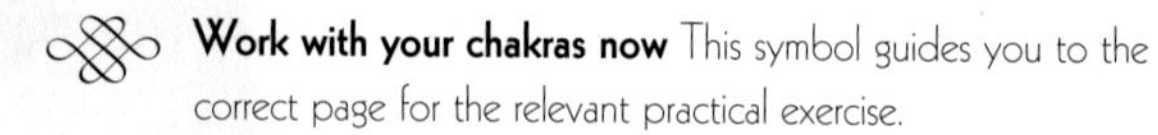

Work with your chakras now This symbol guides you to the correct page for the relevant practical exercise.

I'm not quite there yet If you don't yet feel confident about doing the exercise, this symbol gives suggestions for ways to revise and prepare yourself.

Optional advanced exercise This symbol guides you to the relevant page for more advanced work.

Work with the CD now This symbol tells you when to turn to the CD and which track to select. If you would like to follow the script, turn to the pages indicated.

Subtle energy and the chakras

This workshop-in-a-book experience has been specially designed to lead you step-by-step into a deeper understanding of chakra energy. It is different from an academic course, because you will be asked to familiarize yourself with your own chakras by first reading the written material and then undertaking various exercises. This practical work is essential to appreciate the subtleties of chakras and maintain wellness in a holistic way. You will also be asked to sense the condition and balance of your own chakras and to record this on one of the 'body outline pages' (see page 35 for an example). In addition, each chapter has journal space enabling you to keep notes about your progress. These holistic health teachings will support your realization that you are more than just a physical body. Science can now measure the body's electromagnetic field, which in turn has an even finer, more subtle energy field stretching out as far as 10 m (30 ft), called the aura. This is part of your life-force energy system and is regarded as a 'rainbow of light' – indeed, ancient Indian yogis (dedicated practitioners of yoga) called the chakras 'wheels of light', and this is a very good way to envisage them.

Energy transmission points

Energy is received and transmitted through our chakras. They draw information through a fine network of bio-energy lines called nadis (see page 28). Examples of energy transmission are: a crowd of people in a supermarket feeling stress at the checkout; euphoria at a wedding celebration; or sharing happiness with another person. Where did that energetic feeling come from, and how was it picked up? It is not just something we are hearing or seeing, but *sensing* with all parts of our energy body, comprising the aura and chakras. In Nature, our chakras communicate with all life around, opening us to the natural flow of Creation. Water is affected by our thoughts and emotions, and trees 'talk' to each other, sharing information about soil conditions, predators, rainfall and perhaps even the human beings walking beneath them.!

From the moment we are born, our chakras are concerned with survival and basic instincts, yet simultaneously they remind us that we are Children of Light. All life on this planet is sustained by solar light and spiritual Light (with a capital letter), within the electromagnetic spectrum of colour that is sometimes described as the '49th octave of vibration'.

My aura and luminous body

It is important to understand your aura when studying the chakras. The aura is a fluid, fluctuating, egg-shaped energy field surrounding your physical body with different layers of light energy. Beginning closest to your physical body, these layers are called:

- **Etheric Body:** a holographic energy body that interfaces with the physical body
- **Astral or Emotional Body**: a template of the body, and possibly a place to hold your personality beyond death
- **Lower Mental Body**
- **Higher Mental Body**
- **Spiritual Body**: an energy template for the Etheric Body
- **Causal Body**: a repository for lifetimes of experience
- **Ketheric Body**: your link to superconsciousness and Divine Mind.

These layers coexist because they all have different energetic frequencies. Just as communication signals for cellphones, television and radio don't get mixed up with each other, so the layers of your auric body are separately defined.

Back in 1908–14 a doctor in London, Dr Walter Kilner, developed a chemically coated screen that enabled the aura to be seen by anyone, without the faculty of clairvoyance. We have progressed a great deal since then, with the ability to record energies on very sensitive instruments. We now know that the chakras interpenetrate the auric layers, bringing information energy-flows through our auras – even from deep space – into our bodies. Informational energy also goes back out from our bodies, so we are in two-way communication.

The aura of every human, animal, microbe, plant, tree, stone and crystal vibrates in harmony with the cosmic and elemental energies of Earth, Water, Fire, Air and Spirit. When we are with a crowd of people or walk in a forest of tall trees, our energy fields mingle. We are part of a greater 'field of life', constantly interacting with our surroundings and even extending throughout the cosmos, since biophysicists affirm that all matter is interconnected in the Quantum Field.

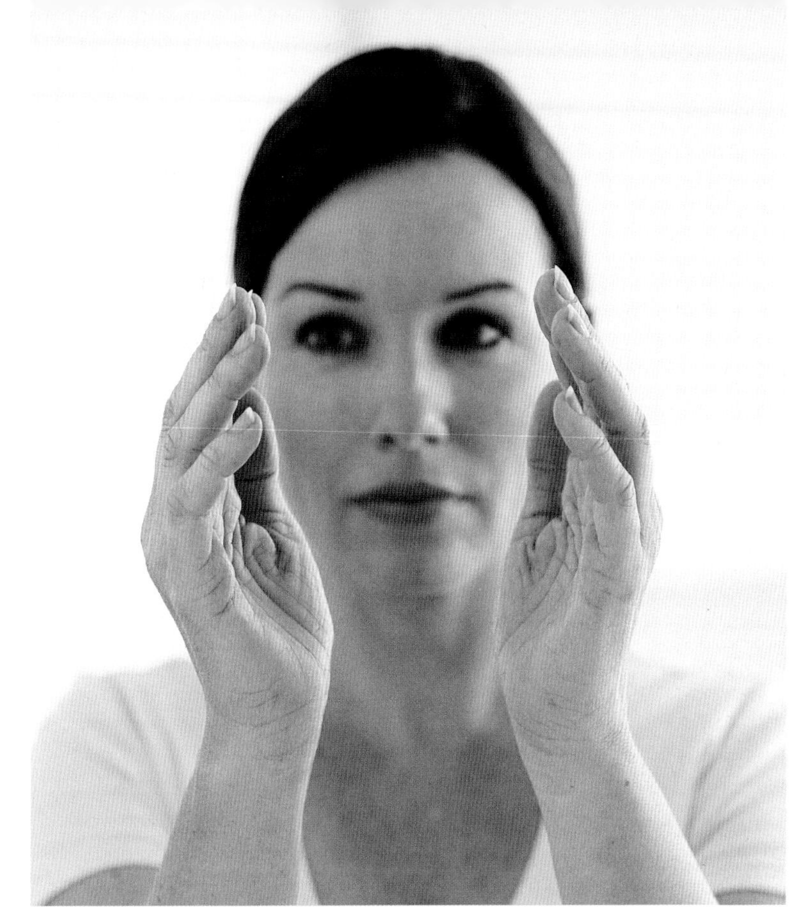

Seeing the aura

You may like to try the following way of seeing your own aura. Sit in a slightly darkened room and rub your hands vigorously together. Then stretch your arms out in front of you, with your fingertips curving toward each other, but not quite touching. Against a dark background, look to a point *beyond* your fingertips, without staring and with a 'soft' gaze. Most people will see very fine lines of light, or colourless, luminous auric streamers, moving from and between their fingers. This is the first and most visible part of your aura.

My seven chakras

Chakras focus the energetic forces of life within our bodies. They are situated within the auric field as swirling masses of colour that interact with our physical bodies at the front, as well as at the back through the spine. They relate particularly to the wellness of our endocrine system (the ductless glands), our central nervous system and spinal fluid. These are the seven main chakras, or power centres, with their associated body areas, starting from the base of the spine:

- **Root or Base Chakra/Muladhara** Associated with the most solid parts of the body, such as the bones, teeth and nails; also with the gonads, anus, rectum, colon, prostate gland, blood and blood cells.
- **Sacral Chakra/Svadisthana** Associated with the pelvis, kidneys and the production of adrenaline; also with the bladder and body liquids: blood, lymph, gastric juices and sperm.
- **Solar Plexus Chakra/Manipura** Associated with the lower back, digestive system, liver, spleen, gall bladder, pancreas and the production of insulin.
- **Heart Chakra/Anahata** Associated with the heart, the upper back and general function of the lungs, blood and air circulation. There is another chakra close to the Heart Chakra, which is linked to the thymus gland and lymphatic system, called the Thymus Chakra.
- **Throat Chakra/Vishuddha** Associated with the throat, neck, thyroid and parathyroid glands, ears, windpipe and the upper parts of the lungs.
- **Third Eye (Brow) Chakra/Ajna** – Associated with the face, nose, sinuses, ears, eyes and brain functions (including the pituitary gland, cerebellum and central nervous system).
- **Crown Chakra/Sahasrara** Mainly associated with the cerebrum and pineal gland (which is sensitive to light levels), thus affecting the entire body; linked to the production of cerebral spinal fluid.